Lecture Notes on Midwifery

For Student Midwives
and Medical Students

by
T F Redman
TD MB ChB FRCS(Edin) FRCOG
*Formerly Senior Clinical Lecturer in Obstetrics
and Gynaecology, University of Leeds
Formerly Consultant Obstetrician and
Gynaecologist,
Leeds (St James's) University Hospital*

Fourth Edition

1985   **WRIGHT** Bristol

Published by   John Wright & Sons Ltd, Techno House, Redcliffe Way, Bristol BS1 6NX, England.

First edition, 1958
Second edition, 1966
Third edition, 1975
Student edition, 1977
Fourth edition, 1985

British Library Cataloguing in Publication Data
Redman, T. F.
    Lecture notes on midwifery: for student midwives and medical students.—4th ed.
1. Obstetrics
I. Title
618.2   RG524

ISBN 0 7236 0812 1

Typeset by   Severntype Repro Services Ltd, Market Street, Wotton-under-Edge, Glos.

Printed in   John Wright & Sons (Printing) Ltd,
Great Britain by   at The Stonebridge Press, Bristol BS4 5NU

Preface to the Fourth Edition

Once more the passage of time, with the inevitable change and progress in some aspects of Obstetrics, has made a new edition a matter of some urgency: the fields of antenatal diagnosis, sonography and management of labour in particular, have changed and expanded considerably.

As before, the work is designed to save medical students and student midwives the boring and distracting task of note-taking during a lecture, as well as assisting the lecturer in its preparation and delivery.

Recent advances have been given much more detailed treatment, for textbooks all tend to be inadequate in these areas, whereas with the more time-honoured material only outline headings are required and the textbook can be used to expand these if required. The section on 'Antenatal Diagnosis of Fetal Abnormalities' is an example requiring such extended treatment.

I have received considerable help from some of my colleagues in the way of discussion in order to clarify and crystallize some of the more controversial points, and in particular I would like to acknowledge the kind assistance given in this way by Professor D. C. A. Bevis and Mr H. N. Macdonald. I would also like to thank my secretary, Miss Hollie Jarvis, for her patience and skill in making sense out of my manuscript.

Preface to the First Edition

Throughout the country at the various training schools where pupil midwives are preparing for their First Examination, approved lecturers in obstetrics are delivering a minimum of thirty-three lectures every six months. It is to cover this course of lectures that the present notes were designed. Some lecturers may prefer to prepare their own notes and for their pupils this book is superfluous, but many busy consultant obstetricians might be glad of a ready-made lecture summary to offer their pupils. It is not intended in any way to replace a textbook which will be required for wider reading and to provide illustrations.

The material included here is strictly that which would fall within the province of the obstetrician and does not attempt to cover the lectures of paediatrician and anaesthetist, nor some of the more practical and purely nursing matters which would fall to the lot of the sister tutor. So far as possible only generally accepted views have been quoted, although recent ideas have been given in preference to more classic ones where evidence appears to be strong enough to justify this. However, so many controversial points exist in obstetrics that for simplicity's sake dogmatic statements may have been made in places where reasoned discussion might have been more applicable. On such occasions the author has no alternative but to quote his own views while fully prepared to accept Cromwell's plea to 'think it possible you may be mistaken'.

The lectures are arranged in two self-contained parts; either section can be given before the other without loss of continuity. This is to overcome the difficulty of dealing with a new intake of people every three months, which means that alternate 'schools' must always begin in the middle of the course.

A good written answer in an examination is always made still better by a relevant sketch. A list is appended of the more important illustrations, a number of which it would profit the pupil to be able to draw from memory. These illustrations, and many others which the lecturer might choose, are a vital accompaniment to a lecture course—in the form of wall charts, blackboard sketches, or lantern slides prepared from textbooks.

The modern pupil midwife has so much highly technical knowledge to absorb during her off-duty time from an arduous day on the ward that any device which helps her in this task is only too welcome. It is hoped that this little work may be of some small assistance to her in preparing for her Part I CMB examination.

Although these notes were planned initially to supply the needs of pupil midwives, it is hoped that the book will give some help to those medical students who find tabulated knowledge a useful adjunct to the conventional textbook.

In a work of this sort help will have been received, consciously or unconsciously, from a large number of teachers, from reference books and original articles—too numerous to list. To one teacher, however, the author would like to record his thanks: that is to the late Professor D. Dougal, of Manchester, whose wonderfully clear lecture notes will be remembered by all his students. It is the memory of the immense assistance those notes gave when preparing for examinations, as well as their value for reference later on, which stimulated the production of this book.

Thanks must also be given to the Leeds (A) Group Hospital Management Committee for their assistance in producing the original duplicated sets of notes and in particular to Miss Margaret Garside, whose hard work and skill produced the clarity of lay-out.

The figures for Maternal Deaths in Leeds, tabulated under the Chapter on Pre-eclampsia, were kindly supplied by Professor I. G. Davies, Medical Officer of Health for Leeds.

November, 1958   TFR

Contents

Part 1 **Pregnancy and its Complications**

Part 2   Labour and the Puerperium

List of Suggested Illustrations

*   Those marked with an asterisk are illustrations which the student should be able to reproduce diagrammatically from memory.

Part 1

Pregnancy and its Complications

Part 2

Labour and the Puerperium

Part 1
Pregnancy and
its Complications

Anatomy of Pelvic Organs and Breast

GENERAL LAY-OUT OF PELVIC ORGANS
(*Figs.* 1, 2)

Structures in the sagittal plane from before,
backwards:
1. Bladder and urethra.
2. Uterus and vagina.
3. Rectum and anal canal.

PELVIC FLOOR MUSCLES (*Figs.* 3–5)

The Pelvic Diaphragm

These muscles are covered by a layer of pelvic
fascia in both upper and lower surfaces.

Levator Ani. Divided into two parts:
1. *Pubococcygeus.* The most important pelvic
floor support.
Origin. From the back of the superior pubic
ramus.
Insertion. The *anterior fibres* of each muscle
unite behind the bladder neck, vagina and anal
canal successively, forming a series of *muscle
slings* which hold these structures upwards and
forwards. Some fibres run actually into their
walls, merging with the intrinsic musculature.
Rupture of these muscle slings at childbirth
may lead to stress incontinence and prolapse
later in life.

3

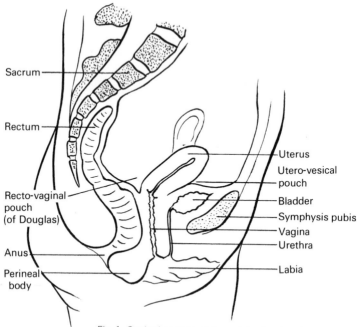

Fig. 1. Sagittal section of the pelvis showing the relationship of the organs.

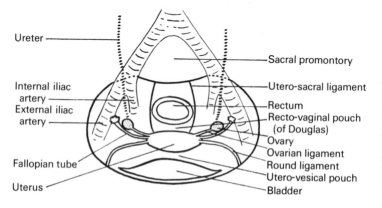

Fig. 2. View of the pelvic organs from above.

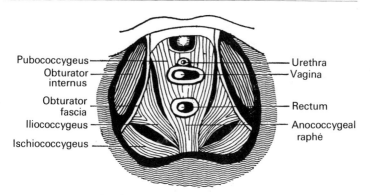

Pubococcygeus
Obturator internus
Obturator fascia
Iliococcygeus
Ischiococcygeus

Urethra
Vagina
Rectum
Anococcygeal raphé

Fig. 3. Muscles of the pelvic floor from above.

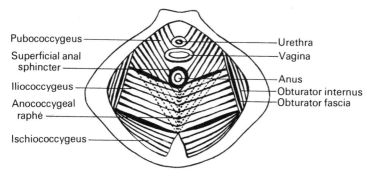

Pubococcygeus
Superficial anal sphincter
Iliococcygeus
Anococcygeal raphé
Ischiococcygeus

Urethra
Vagina
Anus
Obturator internus
Obturator fascia

Fig. 4. Pelvic floor muscles from below.

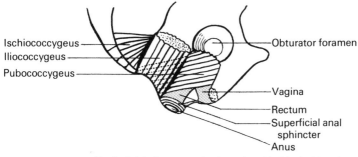

Ischiococcygeus
Iliococcygeus
Pubococcygeus

Obturator foramen
Vagina
Rectum
Superficial anal sphincter
Anus

Fig. 5. Pelvic floor muscles from the side (the ischium has been removed).

The *remaining fibres* from each side unite in the midline to form a tendinous band, the *anococcygeal raphè*, which runs from the anus in front to the tip of the coccyx posteriorly.

2. *Iliococcygeus.* A thin muscle.

Origin. From the 'white line' across the obturator fascia. This fascia runs across the obturator internus muscle on the side wall of the pelvis, covering in the obturator foramen. The 'white line' runs from the pubis anteriorly to the ischial spine posteriorly; it is a tendinous arch.

Insertion. The fibres of each muscle meet in the midline in the *anococcygeal raphè* lying below and overlapped by the pubococcygeus.

Ischiococcygeus. Also known as the 'coccygeus'.

Origin. From the ischial spine.

Insertion. Into the lateral margin of the coccyx and the last piece of the sacrum. It lies on the sacrospinous ligament.

Perineal Muscles (*Fig.* 6)

Deep Transverse Muscle of the Perineum. Between layers of triangular ligament.

The fibres surrounding the urethra are called the 'compressor urethrae muscle'.

Superficial Group. Lying superficially to the triangular ligament.

1. *Ischiocavernosus* (erector clitoridis)
2. *Bulbocavernosus* (sphincter vaginae)
3. *Superficial Transverse Muscle of the Perineum*
4. *Superficial Anal Sphincter.*

} Form a triangle.

PELVIC PERITONEUM

Traced in the Sagittal Plane

Anterior Abdominal Wall. Parietal peritoneum.

Bladder. Firmly adherent to fundus but lies

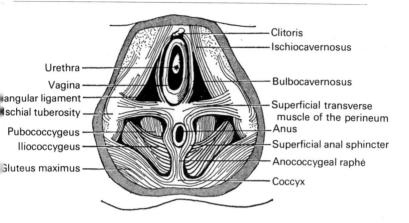

Fig. 6. Perineal muscles.

loosely over the cave of Retzius. Is now called 'visceral peritoneum'.
Uterovesical Pouch. Shallow.
Uterus. Firmly attached all over, except on the lower segment anteriorly, immediately above its reflection from the bladder.
Pouch of Douglas. Deep, and lies close to the posterior vaginal fornix.
Rectum. Firmly attached.
Sacrum. Becomes parietal peritoneum again.

Disposition as seen from above	**Folds** 1. *Uterosacral Fold.* Contains the uterosacral ligament. 2. *Broad 'Ligament'.* Contains the parametrium. **Pouches and Fossae** 1. *Pouch of Douglas.* 2. *Pararectal Fossae.* 3. *Uterovesical Pouch.* 4. *Paravesical Fossae.*

PELVIC CELLULAR TISSUE

Fibromuscular tissue.

Pelvic Fascia (*Fig.* 7)	**Visceral Layer.** Covers all the organs. **Parietal Layer.** Covers the side walls of the pelvis (including the obturator internus muscle and the muscles of the pelvic floor).
Condensations of Pelvic Cellular Tissue running from the Parietes to the Viscera	**Uterosacral Ligaments** **Parametrium and Paravaginal Tissue** (paracolpos).
Remaining Space	The remaining space deep to the pelvic peritoneum and alongside the viscera is filled in by *loose areolar tissue.*

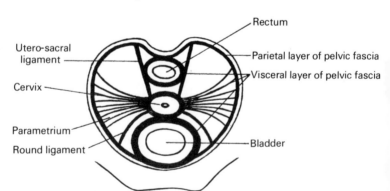

Fig. 7. Pelvic fascia and cellular tissue.

ORGANS

Uterus

Size. $7 \cdot 5 \times 5 \times 2 \cdot 5$ cm. Walls $1 \cdot 5$–2 cm. (External dimensions $2 \cdot 5$ cm greater after pregnancy.)

Parts of Uterus
1. *Body or Corpus* (upper two-thirds of the adult uterus)
a. The corners are called the *cornua* (singular, *cornu*).
b. Attached to each cornu are:
  i. Round ligament ⎫ From
  ii. Fallopian tube ⎬ before
  iii. Ovarian ligament ⎭ backwards.
c. The part above the level of the tubes is called the *fundus.*
2. *Neck or Cervix* (lower one-third of the adult uterus)
a. Two Parts
  i. Vaginal portion.
  ii. Supravaginal portion.
b. Two Openings
  i. Internal os.
  ii. External os.
c. Cervical Canal. Spindle-shaped.
3. *Isthmus*
a. Between corpus and cervix proper: it represents the upper one-third of the naked-eye cervix.
b. Differs from the cervix proper in being lined by an epithelium resembling the endometrium of the corpus, i.e. *anatomically* it appears to be the upper part of the cervix, *histologically* its lining resembles the body of the uterus.
c. Limits: (1) Upper, *anatomical internal os.*
          (2) Lower, *histological internal os.*
d. Function. To form the *lower uterine segment.*

Shape of Uterus
1. *External.* Pear-shaped.

2. *Cavity.* Triangular. Flattened anteroposteriorly, the front and back walls being in contact.

3. The corpus is usually angled forwards on the cervix, i.e. it is *anteflexed.* In some women, however, it is angled backwards, i.e. *retroflexed.*

Relations
1. *Anterior*
a. Uterovesical pouch (and its contents).
b. Bladder.
c. Anterior vaginal fornix.
2. *Posterior*
a. Pouch of Douglas (and its contents).
b. Rectum.
c. Posterior vaginal fornix.
3. *Lateral*
a. Fallopian tubes, ovarian and round ligaments.
b. Broad ligament with the contained parametrium and paracolpos.
c. Lateral vaginal fornices.
d. Ureter.
e. Uterine artery and vein.
4. *Superior.* Coils of bowel.
5. *Inferior.* The vagina. The uterus as a whole is usually *anteverted,* i.e. it is angled forwards on the vagina. the cervix pointing backwards of the vaginal axis.

Structure (from without inwards)
1. *a.* The corpus is covered by a serous or peritoneal layer.
   b. The vaginal portion of the cervix has an outer layer of squamous epithelium.
2. *Visceral Pelvic Fascia* over the uterus and runs down continuously on the vagina.
3. *Muscular Layer*
a. *External Layer.* Longitudinal fibres.
b. *Middle Layer.* Interlacing fibres (main layer).
c. *Internal Layer.* Circular fibres.
   N.B. The corpus is very muscular, the

cervix proper largely fibrous: the isthmus occupies an intermediate position.

4. *Mucosal Layer or Endometrium*

a. Corpus. (i) Low columnar and ciliated cells; (ii) Simple tubular glands, with a tortuous course, which vary with the phase of the menstrual cycle; (iii) Supported by a submucosal layer or *stroma.*

b. Cervix. (i) High palisade epithelium on surface; (ii) Compound racemose glands; (iii) No submucosa.

c. Isthmus. Like the corpus, but with a narrower stroma.

Uterine Attachments

1. *Static Supports*

a. Parametrium and paracolpos. Also called:
(i) Cardinal ligaments of the uterus;
(ii) Transverse cervical ligaments;
(iii) Mackenrodt's ligaments.

b. Uterosacral ligaments.

2. *Dynamic Supports.* Muscles of the pelvic diaphragm.

3. *Other Attachments*

a. Pelvic Fascia. (i) Runs from the outer surface of the uterus on to the outer surface of the vagina without a break: (ii) Serves to anchor the uterus to the pelvis during late pregnancy and labour.

b. Round Ligaments. May help to hold the uterus forward but are not important.

c. Peritoneal Folds. No supporting or anchoring function: (i) Broad 'ligaments';
(ii) Uterosacral folds.

Causes of Prolapse

a. Predisposing Cause. Tearing the pelvic floor muscles at childbirth.

b. Precipitating Cause. Atrophy of static supports, and of remaining muscle, with age.

c. Adjuvant Causes. (i) An inherent tendency;
(ii) Factors producing raised intra-abdominal pressure, e.g. an occupation involving physical strain, chronic cough, obesity, intra-abdominal tumour, etc.

Blood Supply and Venous Drainage (*see* pp. 19, 20)
1. *Uterine Artery and Vein.*
2. *Ovarian Artery and Vein.*

Lymphatic Drainage
1. From cervix to *iliac lymph glands.*
2. From corpus to *para-aortic lymph glands.*

Attitude of the Uterus. Usually the uterus is *anteflexed* and *anteverted* (*see above*), but in 20% of the female population it lies in a backward position, i.e. *retrodisplacement of the uterus* (q.v.).

Fallopian Tubes

Portions of the Tube
1. *Interstitial or Uterine Part.* 1·5–2 cm.
2. *Isthmus.* Inner one-third of tube.
3. *Ampulla.* Outer two-thirds of tube.

Length. 10–11·5 cm.

Abdominal Opening Surrounded by *Fimbriae.*

Structure
1. Serous coat.
2. Muscle layer.
3. Mucosa. Thrown into folds called *plicae.*

Ovary

Size. 4 × 1·5 cm.

Relations (*Fig.* 8)
1. Attached to the posterior layer of the broad ligament by its *hilum.*
2. Attached to uterine cornu by the *ovarian ligament.*
3. The outer end is in contact with the *fimbrial end of the tube.*
4. Posterolaterally lies the *peritoneal fossa* in which the ovary nestles between the bifurcating branches of the common iliac vessel, i.e. the internal and external iliacs.

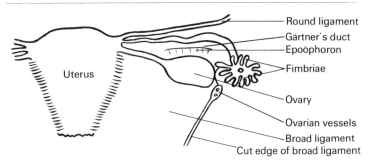

Fig. 8. Relationship of tube and ovary.

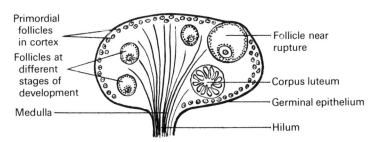

Fig. 9. Section of normal ovary (showing, diagrammatically, various stages of follicular development).

Structure (from without inwards)
1. Germinal epithelium (continuous with peritoneum).
2. Tunica albuginea (dense fibrous tissue).
3. Cortex (stroma containing the follicles).
4. Medulla (smooth muscle and fibrous tissue).
5. Hilum (structure like the medulla).

The Follicles (*Fig.* 9)
1. *Primordial Follicles*
a. Seventy thousand present in fetal ovarian cortex.
b. Structure. (i) Large central *egg-cell*; (ii) Layer of *granulosa cells* (corona radiata) surrounds this.

2. *Graafian Follicles* (begin to form from 36 weeks of intra-uterine life).
Structure:
a. Central *egg-cell.*
b. Granulosa cells split to form a cavity containing liquor folliculi.
c. Theca interna.
d. Theca externa.
Maturation (begins at puberty):
a. Eight to ten follicles may ripen at one time, but only 1 or 2 rupture.
b. The liquor folliculi increases; the follicle swells and moves towards the surface of the ovary.
c. When fully ripe it measures 1 cm in diameter.
Rupture: The ovum is shed into the peritoneal cavity.
3. *Corpus Luteum*
a. Arises from the remains of the ruptured follicle.
b. Measures about 1·5 cm in diameter when fully developed.
c. Begins to degenerate just before the next period (unless a pregnancy occurs).
d. Final form is a *corpus albicans* produced after some weeks by a process of fibrosis.

Epoöphoron and Paroöphoron

These are vestigial structures between the layers of the broad ligament near the ovary. They correspond to the vasa efferentia of the testis. These vestigial tubules enter *Gärtner's duct* which corresponds to the vas deferens of the male.

Vagina

1. *Length.* 10 cm.
2. *Disposition*
a. Upper end receives the vaginal portion of the *cervix,* forming the *vaginal fornices* (left, right, anterior and posterior).
b. Lower end is narrowed by the *hymen* (if present) where it communicates with the exterior via the *vaginal introitus.*

c. The cervix enters the vagina at an angle open forward, if the uterus is in a position of anteversion.

d. The vaginal cavity is really a transverse slit, the anterior and posterior walls being in contact.

3. *Relations*

a. Anterior
  i. Bladder (upper half).
  ii. Urethra (lower half).

b. Posterior
  i. Pouch of Douglas (upper third).
  ii. Rectum (middle third).
  iii. Perineal body (lower third).

c. Lateral
  i. Ureter (close to the lateral fornix).
  ii. Uterine and vaginal vessels.
  iii. Paracolpos.
  iv. Pelvic diaphragm (2·5 cm inside vaginal introitus).

d. Superior
Uterus.

e. Inferior
Introitus.

4. *Structure*

a. Visceral layer of pelvic fascia. Continuous with that covering the uterus.

b. Muscle Layer.

c. Vaginal epithelium (squamous or stratified).

5. *Physiology of the Vagina*

a. It is very distensible due to:
  i. Muscular walls.
  ii. Numerous folds called 'rugae'.

b. Its reaction is *acid* which protects it from infection by most pyogenic organisms. The acid is lactic acid, produced from the glycogen of the vaginal wall cells by the action of Döderlein's bacillus—a normal inhabitant of the healthy vagina. The vaginal deposits of glycogen are brought about by oestrogen from the ovary.

c. It is moist from the following sources:
  i. Mucus from the cervical glands.
  ii. A mucoid secretion from Bartholin's glands.

iii. A watery transudate from the vaginal wall, which has no glands.

d. The mucus output from the cervix is affected by oestrogens and increases under the following circumstances, often bringing the girl or woman to the gynaecologist complaining of 'discharge'. It is important to realize that on most of these occasions all that is necessary is to explain what has occurred, offer reassurance and perhaps to advise her to intensify her usual toilet measures.

i. At the menarche (it is usually the girl's mother who is worried).

ii. During pregnancy (*see* Cervical leucorrhoea in Chapter 4, 'Vaginal Discharge'). This usually persists to some degree when the pregnancy is over.

iii. When on oral contraceptives.

iv. In association with some change in the menstrual flow or cycle.

v. Sometimes with no obvious associated condition.

N.B. The cervical mucoid output is usually cyclic in amount, i.e. it increases during the few days leading up to the period or it may have a mid-cycle peak.

Vulva

Anatomical Parts

Labia majora	Urinary meatus
Mons veneris	Vaginal introitus
Labia minora	Hymen
Clitoris and its prepuce	Bartholin glands
Vestibule	Perineal body

Nerve Supply

1. *Internal Pudendal Nerve*

a. Source. The pudendal plexus (S2, 3, 4).

b. Course. Similar to the internal pudendal artery (*see* p. 20).

c. Terminal Branches. (i) Perineal nerve. (ii) Dorsal nerve of clitoris.

2. *Posterior Cutaneous Nerve of Thigh—Perineal Branch.*

Reaches the surface near the ischial tuberosity and is distributed to the labium majorus.
3. *Ilio-inguinal Nerve.* Branches are distributed to mons veneris and upper part of labium majorus.

Blood Supply from the internal pudendal artery.

Lymphatic Drainage. Mainly to the femoral and inguinal lymph glands, but some drainage from the clitoral area directly to the external iliac glands.

Ureter

Abdominal Course. 15 cm from renal pelvis to pelvic brim.

Pelvic Course. 10 cm from pelvic brim to bladder.
1. Enters the pelvis by crossing the bifurcation of the *common iliac artery* where it lies in the floor of the *ovarian fossa.*
2. Runs downwards and forwards on the side wall of the pelvis to the back of the broad ligament.
3. Turns inwards towards the lateral vaginal fornix and runs along the posterior leaf of the broad ligament.
4. Runs forwards to enter the bladder 2 cm from the cervix where it is crossed by the *uterine vessels.*

Bladder

Average Capacity is about 400 ml.

Relations
1. *Base*
a. Uterus (lower segment).
b. Vagina (upper part).
2. *Inferolateral Surfaces*
a. Pubis.
b. Cave of Retzius.
c. Pelvic diaphragm.
3. *Superior Surface (covered by peritoneum)*
a. Uterovesical pouch.

b. Uterus.
c. Coils of small bowel, etc.

Structure
1. *Muscular Layer.* Thick smooth muscle.
2. *Mucous Layer*
a. In many folds when empty.
b. Consists of *transitional epithelium.*
3. *The Trigone.* A smooth triangular area in the base of the bladder, seen when it is opened.
a. The angles of the triangle are the two ureteric and the internal urethral orifices.
b. The interureteric bar of muscle runs between the two ureteric orifices.

Urethra

Length. 4 cm.

Relations. Lies on the lower half of the anterior vaginal wall.

Structure
1. *Muscular Layer.*
2. *Mucous Layer* (squamous epithelium).

Urinary Control (Prof. J. A. Gosling)*
Anatomy
a. Bladder neck (i) Considerable *elastic tissue* in and around the bladder neck and proximal urethra. (ii) No muscle sphincter exists in this area.
b. Mid urethra (the zone of maximal closure pressure). Circular striated muscle fibres—the *'external sphincter'.*
c. Distal urethra (i) *Sling of pubococcygeus* of levator ani (just distal to the external sphincter). (ii) The lower urethra is devoid of any significant sphincter.
Factors producing continence
a. Passive elastic resistance of urethral wall.
b. External sphincter—mainly provides occlusion at rest.

*The Incontinent Woman. Proc. Meet. R. Coll. Obstet. Gynaecol. Feb. 1981.

c. Pubococcygeus—provides additional occlusive force during stress.
d. The position of the bladder neck above the pelvic floor allows intra-abdominal pressure to constrict the upper urethra.

Pelvic Colon

Extent. From the left sacro-iliac joint to the front of the third sacral vertebra.

Length. 40 cm.
Completely surrounded by *peritoneum.*

Rectum

Extent. From the front of the third sacral vertebra to the *pelvic diaphragm.*

Length. 12 cm.

Anal Canal

Extent. From the *pelvic diaphragm* to the *anus.*

Length. 4 cm.

Relations
1. *Anterior.* The perineal body.
2. *Posterior.* The anococcygeal body.
3. *Lateral.* The fat of the ischiorectal fossa.

BLOOD SUPPLY OF THE PELVIC ORGANS

Internal Iliac or Hypogastric Vessels

	Anterior Branches		*Posterior Branches*
1.	*Visceral*		
	(Some)	Superior vesical	
	(Usually)	Uterine	
	(Inherit)	Inferior vesical (Usually replaced by the vaginal artery in the female)	
	(Money)	Middle haemorrhoidal	

	Anterior Branches		Posterior Branches	
2.	*Somatic*			
	(Others)	Obturator	(Such)	Superior gluteal
	(Inherit)	Internal pudendal	(Is)	Iliolumbar
	(Insanity)	Inferior gluteal	(Life)	Lateral sacral

N.B. Each artery has its companion vein.

Ovarian Vessels

1. *Arteries* arise from the front of the *aorta,* at the level of the kidneys, and approach the ovaries via the *infundibulopelvic ligaments.* (This high origin is because the fetal ovaries develop in the kidney region, later migrating to the pelvis, followed by their blood supply.)
2. *Veins* follow the course of the arteries most of the way, but:
a. The left vein enters the *left renal vein.*
b. The right vein enters the *inferior vena cava.*

Details of Certain Arteries

1. *The Uterine Artery* arises from the anterior branch of the internal iliac artery and runs directly inwards through the parametric tissue to reach the uterus where the corpus meets the cervix. It crosses the ureter on the way 1·5 cm lateral to the uterus. On reaching the uterus it divides into:
a. *A descending* or *cervical branch* (supplies cervix and vagina).
b. *An ascending branch* which runs up the side of the uterus, giving off branches on the way, and ends in terminal branches to:
  i. The uterine fundus.
 ii. The Fallopian tube.
iii. Anastomose with the ovarian artery.
2. *The Internal Pudendal Artery* arises from the anterior branch of the internal iliac artery and leaves the pelvis through the great sciatic foramen, winds around the outside of the ischial spine, and then courses across the inner aspect of the ischium (and the obturator internus muscle), 4 cm above the ischial tuberosity, in Alcock's canal. It reaches the

perineal region and supplies the anal canal, vulval structures, and the lower part of the vagina; it ends in the clitoris.

MAMMARY GLANDS

Position

The glands are developed as modified sebaceous glands and therefore lie in the *superficial fascia.* They lie over the *pectoralis major* muscle.

Extent

Vertically. Second to 6th rib inclusive (5 ribs).

Horizontally. Side of the sternum to the midaxillary line. *N.B.* Axillary tail of Spence.

Nipple

1. Lies in the 4th intercostal space, 10 cm from the midline.
2. Has 20 lactiferous ducts opening on it, each from one lobe.
3. Its base is encircled by *smooth* muscle fibres which are concerned in causing erection of the nipple.

Areola

1. Has no subcutaneous tissue.
2. Small projections occur which are sebaceous glands and are called *Montgomery's tubercles.* These produce a greasy substance which lubricates the skin of the nipple.

Architecture of the Gland (*Fig.* 10)

Composed of glandular and fatty tissue.
1. *Lobes.* Twenty of them formed by 20 radiating fibrous septa. Each lobe contains (from the nipple outwards):
a. Lactiferous duct.
b. Ampulla. A dilated portion of the duct just below the areola which acts as a milk reservoir.
c. Lobules. Like a bunch of grapes around the lactiferous ducts.
2. Each *lobule* consists of a cluster of rounded sacs called *alveoli* or *acini.*

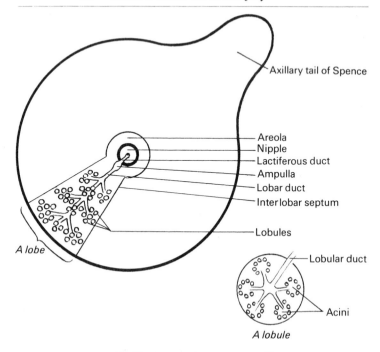

Fig. 10. Section of normal breast (diagrammatic).

Arterial Supply	**1.** *Internal Mammary.* Anterior perforating arteries of 2nd, 3rd and 4th spaces. **2.** *External Mammary.* From the lateral thoracic branch of the axillary artery. **3.** *Intercostal.* Lateral branches of 2nd, 3rd and 4th spaces.
Venous Drainage	A *venous plexus* forms beneath the *areola.* Large vessels pass from this to the periphery of the gland, ultimately draining into: *a.* The internal mammary vein, *b.* The axillary vein.

Lymphatic Drainage

1. *Overlying skin* (excluding skin of areola and nipple):
a. Outer side—to axillary glands.
b. Upper part—to subclavicular glands.
c. Inner side—to internal mammary glands.
N.B. The skin lymphatics communicate across the midline.

2. *Breast Parenchyma* and the *skin of the Areola and Nipple:*
a. Most of the drainage is into the *subareolar lymph plexus.* Two trunks (one from the inner and one from the outer side) drain this plexus. Each trunk receives a vessel direct from the breast parenchyma. The two trunks unite to form a single one which goes to the *axillary lymph glands.*
b. The *upper part* of the mamma sends one vessel direct to the *subclavicular glands* through the pectoralis major.
c. The *inner part* of the mamma communicates with the internal mammary glands. and thence to the *lymphatics of the opposite breast.*
d. The *lower and inner quadrant* of the breast communicates via the rectus sheath and linea alba with the *subperitonial lymph plexus.*

2 Physiology of Pregnancy

FEMALE SEX CYCLE

Ovarian Cycle	*Menstrual or Uterine Cycle*
Follicular Phase (1st–14th day): Maturation of the Graafian follicle up to and including rupture.	*Menstrual Phase* (1st–4th day): Breakdown of endometrium through the spongy layer.
	Proliferative Phase (5th–14th day): i. Build up of the endometrium from the basal layer. ii. The endometrial glands are straight and regular.
Luteal Phase (15th–28th day): Development of the corpus luteum from the remains of the ruptured follicle. After full activity there follows a gradual process of regression, beginning four days before the next period occurs and extending over many months.	*Secretory Phase* (15th–28th day): i. Further development of the endometrium in preparation for receiving a fertilized ovum. ii. The endometrial glands are tortuous and 'saw-toothed' in outline, the duct cavities being filled with secretion.

ENDOCRINOLOGY

Ovarian Hormones

Oestrogens

1. *Types*

a. Natural: Oestradiol is the most important. Produced commercially as: (i) pellets for implant; (ii) oestradiol benzoate for injection; (iii) oestradiol valerate—given by mouth.

b. Synthetic: Given by mouth.
Ethinyloestradiol (chemically similar to natural oestrogens).
Stilboestrol, dienoestrol (chemically quite different from natural oestrogens).

2. *Sources of Natural Oestrogens*

a. Granulosa and theca interna cells of the Graafian follicle.

b. Placenta.

c. Adrenal cortex.

3. *Functions.* The name oestrogen is given because these substances produce oestrous changes in spayed animals.

a. Produce secondary sex characteristics at puberty, e.g. voice changes, feminine curves, secretion of apocrine glands, soft skin, etc.
N.B. Development of axillary or pubic hair is controlled by androgens, probably of adrenocortical origin.

b. Stimulates growth of genital organs (e.g. the uterus) to some extent in childhood but to a much more marked extent at puberty and pregnancy.

c. Maintains the healthy state of the genital organs during the reproductive period, e.g. the vaginal wall is thick, folded in rugae, and the cells contain glycogen (*see* p. 15). After the menopause this protection is lost.

d. Stimulates the cervical glands to produce watery mucus (*see* pp. 16, 26) which produces fern-like crystals of sodium chloride on drying.

e. Produces the proliferative phase of the endometrium and primes it for progesterone to produce the secretory phase.

f. Sensitizes the muscle of the uterus and Fallopian tube to oxytocin.

g. Produces hypertrophy of the duct system of the mammary glands at puberty and in pregnancy.

h. Controls the output of pituitary hormones. Rising oestrogen output in the first half of the ovarian cycle:

Reduces the output of FSH.

Stimulates the production of LH.

The high level of placental oestrogen in pregnancy antagonizes the output of prolactin.

Progesterone

1. *Sources*

a. Corpus luteum.

b. Placenta.

c. Adrenal cortex.

2. *Functions*

a. Makes the cervical mucus more viscous and abolishes 'ferning'.

b. Produces the secretory phase of the endometrium after priming by oestrogen. This endometrium is in readiness for the fertilized ovum. Withdrawal of oestrogen and progesterone leads to the menstrual period.

c. It is necessary for the continuation of pregnancy, but it is not certain how it acts.

d. Causes slower but stronger contractions of the uterus and Fallopian tubes.

e. Produces hypertrophy of the lobule-alveolar system of the mammary gland, acting in conjunction with oestrogens. New alveolar cells develop during pregnancy.

f. Rising progesterone output in the second half of the ovarian cycle reduces the output of LH.

Pituitary Hormones

Anterior Lobe (Adenohypophysis)

1. *Gonadotrophins*

a. Follicle stimulating hormone (FSH)

Causes development of the follicle up to the point of ovulation and stimulates the granulosa

and theca interna cells to produce oestrogen.
The increasing output of oestrogen then inhibits
further output of FSH.

b. Luteinizing hormone (LH).
Stimulates ovulation and then further output
causes development of the corpus luteum and
the production of progesterone.
The increasing output of progesterone then
inhibits further output of LH.

N.B. A large amount of a similar hormone is
produced by the placenta reaching a maximum
output at about the 12th week of pregnancy.
This substance gives the positive pregnancy
tests (q.v.).

2. *Prolactin*
Closely related to growth hormone and may be
identical with luteotrophic hormone (LTH)
which in animals is necessary for maintenance
of the corpus luteum: there is no evidence for
this action in human physiology.

The *output* increases during pregnancy but
falls during lactation. It is pulsatile.

Actions
a. It is necessary for *lactation.* Its action on
the breast is blocked peripherally in pregnancy
by the placental steroids.

b. It *blocks the action of gonadotrophins*
either directly or through the gonadotrophin
release factor (GnRH or LHRH).

N.B. There are many other hormones from
the anterior lobe of the pituitary affecting
every endocrine gland in the body.

Posterior Lobe (Neurohypophysis)
The two hormones connected with this part of
the pituitary are produced by the hypothalamus
(q.v.) and travel to the posterior lobe of the
pituitary along the axons of the nerves
connecting the two structures. They are stored
in the pituitary to be liberated by nerve
impulses from the hypothalamus.

1. *Oxytocin.* Causes uterine muscle to
contract. Marketed as Syntocinon.

2. *Vasopressin* (also known as 'antidiuretic hormone').
Causes blood vessels to contract, but as its effect is so marked on the coronary vessels of the heart it produces shock.

Hypothalamus

Site
1. Above the pituitary and anatomically continuous with the posterior pituitary.
2. Forms floor of third ventricle.
3. Posterior to optic chiasma.

A Portal Venous System carries blood, and therefore, hormones, from the hypothalamus to the pituitary gland.

Hormones
1. *Luteinizing Hormone Release Hormone* (LHRH) now known as (Gonadotrophin Release Hormone (GnRH))
a. Its release is pulsatile and approximately hourly.
b. It effects the release by the pituitary of both FSH and LH. There is a differential in output of FSH and LH created by the different clearance rates of the two hormones: FSH has a lower clearance rate and therefore, initially, a higher blood level with a given pulse.
2. *Prolactin Inhibitory Factor* (PIF)— probably dopamine.
(Bromocriptine either mimics or stimulates the output of PIF thereby reducing the output of prolactin by the pituitary.)
3. Other release hormones exist, e.g. Growth hormone RH, Thyrotropin RH, Corticotropin RH.

Co-ordination of Ovary, Pituitary and Hypothalamus

1. Early in the follicular phase, the low concentration of oestrogen allows an *increased output of FSH* (positive feedback).
2. With increased output of follicular oestrogen *FSH output is damped down* (negative feedback). The follicle which has become most advanced and will in due course

ovulate can continue to develop without FSH
stimulus.

3. Further increase of oestrogen output from
the developing follicle triggers an *LH surge*
and release of *prostaglandin F 2 α* (positive
feedback). These two factors lead to ovulation.

4. After ovulation:

Oestrogen and progesterone from the corpus luteum
↓ (negative feedback)
Fall in response of ovary to GnRH
↓
Fall in output of FSH and LH
↓
Decay of corpus luteum
↓
Fall in output of oestrogen
↓ (positive feedback)
FSH increase
Development of follicles in next cycle

COITUS, INSEMINATION AND FERTILIZATION

Orgasm

Orgasm is the name given to the crisis of
sexual excitement reached during intercourse.

1. *Female Orgasm* is largely emotional with
the minimum of obvious activity by the genital
organs. Conception can occur without orgasm
in the female.

2. *Male Orgasm,* while also having a large
emotional factor, is accompanied by the
process of *ejaculation.* As this occurs, *seminal
fluid* is deposited in the posterior fornix of the
vagina. A single ejaculate is between 2 and
4·5 ml in volume and should contain not less
than 60000000 *spermatozoa* (the male germ
cell) per ml.

Fertilization

1. *The Ovum,* shed from the follicle into the
peritoneal cavity, enters the Fallopian tube,
being carried there passively by:
a. The constant sweeping movement of the

tubal fimbriae across the surface of the ovary, and

b. A current of peritoneal fluid flowing towards the uterus (produced by the ciliated epithelium lining the tube).

2. *The Spermatozoa,* which are actively motile by means of their tails, swarm up through the uterine cavity to the tube.

3. *Fertilization* occurs in the Fallopian tube, one spermatozoon only fusing with the ovum.

N.B. The ovum probably only survives for a few hours if not fertilized and the spermatozoa only for about a day after insemination. Thus, in each menstrual cycle there is only a period of a day or two during which conception can occur.

DURATION OF PREGNANCY

Two hundred and eighty days from the first day of the last period if the patient has a 28-day cycle.

Two hundred and sixty-six days from the time of ovulation.

N.B. Ovulation is consistently 14 days before the following period, regardless of the length of the cycle.

EMBEDDING OF THE FERTILIZED OVUM

(Occurs between the 5th and 8th day after fertilization)

Decidua Basalis. The endometrium deep to the ovum.

Decidua Capsularis. The endometrium round the ovum.

Decidua Vera. The remaining endometrium.

DEVELOPMENT OF THE OVUM

Ovum

First two weeks.

Morula (a mulberry-like mass).
1. *Embryonic Cell Mass* (central cells).
2. *Trophoblast.*

Blastocyst
1. *Endoderm.* Forms the alimentary canal.
2. *Amnio-embryonic Cavity* (7½ days).
Forms: (*a*) Ectoderm—skin and central
nervous system; (*b*) Amniotic cavity.
3. *Mesoderm* (11½ days). Forms: (*a*) Blood
and blood vessels; (*b*) Muscle; (*c*) Bone; (*d*)
Ligaments; (*e*) All connective tissue in the
body. Also forms the chorion which lines the
trophoblast.

Embryo

3rd to 5th weeks.

Fetus

6th to 40th weeks.

Fetal Length at different periods.
Length in cm = age in lunar months² (up to
and including 5 lunar months)
= age in lunar months × 5 (from
5 lunar months upwards).

Fetal Weight
1. At 28 weeks the fetus weights 1500 g.
2. Thereafter gains 150 g per week.

Fetal Development
1. *At 12 Weeks.* (*a*) All organs are formed
and the fetus is complete; (*b*) The sex is
distinguishable; (*c*) The placenta has formed.
2. *At 28 Weeks.* Said to be 'viable', but a few
survive at less than 28 weeks.
3. *At 36 Weeks.* Nails reach finger-tips.
4. *At 40 Weeks.* Nails project beyond
finger-tips.

FETAL CIRCULATION

Study a wall chart carefully.

Points which differ from the Adult Circulation

1. (*a*) Umbilical *vein* contains *red* blood; (passes towards the fetal heart); (*b*) Umbilical *arteries* contain *blue* blood.

2. The *umbilical vein* runs from the *umbilicus,* past the liver (which it supplies) to the junction with the *portal vein.*

3. The *ductus venosus* runs from the latter point to the *inferior vena cava.*

4. Blood from the *inferior vena cava* is diverted into the *left atrium* by the *Eustachian valve,* passing through the *foramen ovale* in the interauricular septum.

Thence it enters the *left ventricle* and passes into the *aorta.*

5. Blood from the *superior vena cava* is directed into the *right ventricle* by the *Eustachian valve,* passing through the *tricuspid valve.* (It is not certain to what extent the two streams crossing the right atrium mix.)

Thence it enters the *pulmonary artery,* from whence:

a. Some goes to the lungs.

b. Most goes via the *ductus arteriosus* to the thoracic aorta, mixing with the blood coming from the *left ventricle.*

b. The internal iliac arteries continue as the *umbilical arteries* which course up to the *umbilicus.*

Changes occurring at or after Birth

Sequence of Events

1. Clamping of umbilical cord causes the fetal blood CO_2 to rise and O_2 to fall. This leads to gasping respirations (*see below*) and the lungs open up, which also opens up the lung capillary bed so that the blood flows freely from the pulmonary arteries into the lungs whereas before it had been a mere trickle.

2. The rise in oxygen concentration in the blood when respiration is established acts on a sphincter in the ductus arteriosus causing it to contract, thereby restricting blood flow from the pulmonary artery into the aortic arch and forcing it out into the lungs.

3. The free flow of blood into the lungs lowers the pressure on the right side of the heart. Blood previously flowed from the right to the left atrium but now with the fall of pressure on the right side of the heart it would try to reverse its flow were it not for a valvular fold over the foramen ovale which prevents this, being closed by the pressure.

The change from fetal to adult circulation is complete.

Timing of Events

1. 'Physiological' closure occurs as follows:

a. Umbilical arteries and vein at birth.

b. Ductus arteriosus—within 5 minutes of birth.

c. Foramen ovale—within 4 minutes of birth.

d. Ductus venosus—closes between the 6th day and the 6th week.

2. 'Anatomical' closure occurs at a variable and longer interval after birth, if it occurs at all.

FETAL RESPIRATION

1. Towards term the demands of the growing fetus outstrip the rate of development of the placenta so that the respiratory status of the fetus becomes increasingly precarious, resulting in relative anoxia.

2. *The initiation of respiratory movements* depends on a *decreased oxygen supply.* Such anoxia reduces the threshold of the respiratory centre to a level at which the *carbon dioxide* circulating in the fetal blood becomes an effective stimulus.

3. *a. Respiratory movements occur in utero*

in late pregnancy, presumably due to the relative placental insufficiency.

b. Normally such movement is not enough to open up the alveoli. Where, however, a greater degree of intra-uterine anoxia occurs (e.g. in accidental haemorrhage, inco-ordinate action, etc.), gasping movements may take place, liquor amnii, debris, and even infected material being sucked into the lung passages, interfering with respiration at birth and possibly producing intra-uterine pneumonia.

4. *At birth,* the immediate cutting off of the maternal oxygen supply and the rise of the fetal blood carbon dioxide set off normal respiration with expansion of the lung passages by air.

FUNCTIONS OF THE PLACENTA

Respiratory
1. Supply of oxygen.
2. Removal of carbon dioxide.

Nutritive
Supply of the essential food factors.
1. Glucose—to supply energy.
2. Amino acids—to make protein.
N.B. Fats cannot pass the placenta so it may be that fetal fat has to be synthesized from carbohydrate or amino acid.

Excretory
Disposal of waste products, e.g. urea.

Glycogenic
Storage of glycogen ('animal' starch). This is formed from glucose and can be reconverted to that sugar and released again when required for energy production.

Endocrine
Production of certain hormones, including:
1. Oestrogens.
2. Progesterone.

3. Chorionic gonadotrophin ('pituitary-like' hormone).
4. Human chorionic somatomammotrophin (hCS) (formerly known as human placental lactogen (HPL). Similar to pituitary growth hormone. Its function is not clear but estimation of its level in the maternal serum is sometimes used as a test of placental efficiency.

Barrier

Protection against noxious substances. Many harmful substances can pass, however, e.g.:
1. Drugs, e.g. morphine, thalidomide.
2. Antibodies, e.g. anti-Rh.
3. The spirochaete of syphilis.
4. The virus of rubella (*see* p. 135).
It is rare for any other organisms to affect the fetus.

LIQUOR AMNII

Circulation

Production
Mainly a secretion from the amniotic membrane.
N.B. (*a*) In the abnormal fetus with a myelocele, *cerebrospinal fluid* may add to the quantity. (*b*) The bulk of the evidence is against the hypothesis that *fetal urine* plays much part.

Disposal. The fetus *swallows* the liquor and absorbs it from its gastro-intestinal tract. The excess fluid is thus passed back to the mother via the placenta.

Average Quantity. 1–2 litres.

The fluid in the liquor is exchanged completely every 3 hours, according to estimates using radio-isotopes. It is, however, difficult to accept that the fetus could swallow such amounts, which suggests the need for further research. It is probable that the amniotic membrane absorbs as well as secretes the liquor.

Functions

1. Maintenance of an *even temperature.*
2. *Protection* against: (*a*) Blows and shocks; (*b*) Pressure from outside.
3. *Allows free movement* of the fetal parts.
4. *Prevents infection* during labour and flushes out the lower genital tract when the membranes rupture.

N.B. It is doubtful if the classically taught 'fluid wedge' action of the forewaters in dilating the cervix is of any importance, as the presenting part will do the work just as well.

MATERNAL CHANGES IN PREGNANCY

Uterus

1. *Weight* of full term uterus is 1 kg (non-pregnant uterus, nulligravid 45 g, parous 50–70 g).
2. *Measurements* at full term: $30 \times 25 \times 20$ cm. the thickness of the uterine wall decreases towards term, measuring less than 0·5 cm in the latter half of pregnancy.
3. The *muscle fibres* hypertrophy enormously, but some new ones are formed.
4. *Elastic tissue* is laid down and increased in amount.
5. *Blood vessels* become greatly enlarged.
6. The *uterine muscle* becomes increasingly more reactive during pregnancy. *Painless rhythmical contractions* occur from the 4th month onwards and can be elicited or accentuated by palpation.
7. The *lower uterine segment* is formed from the *isthmus* which opens out to become part of the uterine cavity between the 3rd and 4th months of pregnancy. It develops and expands during the latter half of pregnancy, but this process is more marked in labour when at full dilatation the lower segment may be 8 cm wide.

Ovary

1. *Ovulation* ceases.
2. The *corpus luteum* of pregnancy reaches its maximum size at the 4th month and afterwards retrogresses.

Vagina

1. Acquires a *violet coloration* due to increased vascularity.
2. Becomes more *acid.*
3. *Cervical mucus* secretion increases considerably.

Mammary Glands

1. *Increase in size and firmness* due to action of oestrogen and progesterone.
2. *a. Primary areola* becomes more deeply pigmented.
b. A secondary areola may form.
c. Montgomery's tubercles develop.
3. *Colostrum* can be expressed.

Pelvic Joints

These acquire some increased mobility.

Blood Volume

This increases by about 25% in pregnancy. However, the plasma volume increases by more than the red cell volume: this results in a haemodilution with a fall in haemoglobin concentration to 11 g or less per dl. (*See* 'Iron-deficiency Anaemia', p. 41.)

Cardiac Output

The cardiac output increases during pregnancy to between 30 and 50% above the level before pregnancy.

3 Management of Pregnancy

DIAGNOSIS OF PREGNANCY

Probable Symptoms

1. Amenorrhoea.
2. Morning sickness—between 6th and 16th week.
3. Frequency of micturition.
4. Quickening—17th week.

Probable Signs

1. Secretion from the breasts.
2. Uterine enlargements, (*a*) Vaginally at 6–8 weeks, (*b*) Abdominally at 12 weeks.
3. Hegar's sign (softening of the cervix between 6th and 12th week).
4. Vaginal violet coloration—12th week.

Positive Signs

1. Ultrasonography—fetal sac may be seen at 4–4½ weeks (i.e. at the time of the first missed period or half a week later).
   Fetal heart may be seen beating at 6–7 weeks (i.e. 2–3 weeks after the first missed period).
2. Auscultation of the fetal heart—20th week.
3. Ballottement of fetal parts ⎫ Later in
4. Palpation of fetal parts ⎭ pregnancy.

Detection of Chorionic Gonadotrophin in the Urine

Methods
1. *a.* Early morning specimen.
b. Add anti-HCG serum.
c. Test for residual HCG by a *flocculation test* using HCG-coated latex particles or a *haemagglutination inhibition* test using red cells primed with HCG.
N.B. There is little indication for performing these tests when ultrasound is available for:
a. There is a significant false positive rate.
b. There is no indication of viability of the pregnancy.
c. Ultrasound gives an immediate answer.
2. *Radioimmune assay* gives a quantitative estimation, especially for the diagnosis of hydatidiform mole or choriocarcinoma.

Differential Diagnosis

1. Pseudocyesis.
2. Obesity.
3. Ascites.
4. Distended bladder.
5. Ovarian cyst.
6. Fibroids.

HISTORY OF ANTENATAL CARE

Middle of nineteenth century—Burdon (Belfast Lying-in Hospital) advised his students to visit their patients weekly before delivery.

1878—Pinard advised examination of patients during pregnancy to correct transverse lies.

1895—Pinard advocated routine antenatal supervision, and was followed later by Haig Ferguson.

1901—*The first antenatal beds were opened,* Edinburgh Royal Maternity Hospital, due to the enthusiasm of Ballantyne.

1909—*Domiciliary antenatal supervision* was undertaken by nurses in Boston.

1910—*The first antenatal clinic* opened in Adelaide by Wilson.

1911—Antenatal clinic opened in Boston.

1912—Antenatal clinic opened in Sydney.

1913—Domiciliary antenatal service started in Edinburgh.

1915—A year when many antenatal clinics were opened.

Haig Ferguson, opened a clinic in Edinburgh; after a short time taken over by Ballantyne.

Metropolitan Borough of Woolwich opened a municipal clinic.

National League for maternity and Child Welfare (a voluntary body) opened six experimental clinics.

Leeds Babies Welcome Association opened eight clinics.

1918—Maternity and Child Welfare Act (England and Wales) empowered local authorities to establish antenatal clinics and provide other services.

There were 120 clinics open by 1918.

1944—There were 1931 clinics.

OBJECTS OF ANTENATAL CARE

Stress the importance of the promotion of good general health (both mental and physical), as well as the educational side of antenatal care. There is a grave danger in the clinic of laying too much emphasis on the abnormal.

MEDICAL ASPECTS OF ANTENATAL CARE

Detect Certain Associated Diseases which have a bearing on Pregnancy

Major Conditions
1. Anaemia
2. Diabetes and other glycosuria
3. Cardiac disease
4. Urinary infections
5. Nephritis
6. Syphilis
7. Pulmonary tuberculosis
8. Thyrotoxicosis

See immediately below

9. Rubella (*see* p. 135)
10. Thrombo-embolism
11. Essential hypertension (*see* p. 105)

Minor Conditions
1. Varicose veins
2. Heartburn
3. Constipation
4. Haemorrhoids

Dealt with under 'Hygiene of Pregnancy'

5. Vaginal discharges (*see* p. 77).

Anaemia
1. *The Importance of Anaemia in Pregnancy*
a. The anaemic woman will be seriously inconvenienced by the additional physical strain of pregnancy and labour: yet these conditions, being physiological ones, should interfere little with the normal way of life of the healthy person.
b. Anaemia will considerably increase the seriousness of postpartum haemorrhage, should this occur.
c. Recovery from sepsis, or other complications of labour, will be more delayed in the anaemic patient.
2. *Iron-deficiency Anaemia*
a. Factors Involved:
  i. *Hydraemia causing a 10% drop in Hb. Therefore the lower limit of 'normal' in pregnancy can be taken as 11 g/dl.*

N.B. There is some evidence that giving iron preparations prophylactically in pregnancy can prevent this so-called 'physiological anaemia'.
 ii. *Deficient absorption of iron by mouth:* Perhaps due to the achlorhydria of pregnancy.
iii. *Iron deficiency before pregnancy:* The demands of the fetus during pregnancy are not so much greater than the loss of iron due to menstruation before pregnancy as to affect the haemoglobin level to a large extent.

Iron 'Balance Sheet'

Intake (per month)	*Output (per month)*

Iron absorbed from the gut
Poor diet, 70 mg
Good diet, 120 mg
	Before Pregnancy
	Average, 25 mg
	    (Top limit of normal,
	    80 mg
	    Menorrhagia, up to
	    450 mg)

	Pregnant Woman
	Average for the
	    nine months, 100 mg,
	    but half the total
	    demand comes in the
	    last trimester.

Observations: A woman with fairly heavy periods and a poor diet, or with menorrhagia even on a good diet, will be anaemic before pregnancy begins unless she has been taking an iron supplement. A haemoglobin estimation in early pregnancy is vital. It should be repeated at 34 weeks and indeed it may be performed at other visits with advantage if facilities are available. The diagnosis or exclusion of anaemia by pallor of skin or conjunctivitis is impossible.
iv. *Multiple pregnancy:* increased demand.
b. *Iron Therapy:*
 i. *Oral*

	Maintenance	*Treatment*
Ferrous sulphate	200 mg daily	400 mg bd

Always interview the patient with severe anaemia in 7 days to ensure that she has been taking her tablets.

Nausea and vomiting sometimes occur but usually can be avoided if the tablets are taken with food.

N.B. It is always better to give drugs on a once or twice per day dosage unless there is some special reason for more frequent dosage as with antibiotics. It is difficult for the patient to remember frequent dosage—few doctors or nurses can!

ii. *Intramuscular iron* may be ordered when: No oral preparation can be tolerated.

A satisfactory trial with an oral preparation has not provided an adequate response and megaloblastic anaemia has been excluded.

Time is too short to risk a trial with oral iron.

Dosage. For each g/dl of Hb increase required allow 250 mg of iron dextran (Imferon). Give a test dose of 125 mg and the rest by 250 mg on alternate days.

iii. *Total dose infusion.*

Requirement in mg of iron dextran (Imferon) = Hb deficiency in g/dl × 250 + 50%. For example, an Hb deficiency of 4 g/dl would require 1500 mg.

Rate of drip: 10 drops/min for 30 min. If tolerated 45 drops/min.

3. *Megaloblastic Anaemia of Pregnancy. Suspect this condition when:*

i. There is a dramatic fall of haemoglobin during pregnancy or puerperium (in the absence of bleeding anywhere).

ii. An anaemia fails to respond to adequate oral therapy. Confirmation is possible by sternal marrow puncture or by blood folic acid estimation, but this is not necessary in routine work.

Multiple pregnancy has an increased incidence of folic acid deficiency anaemia.

Treatment—Folic acid 5 mg daily. It is reasonable to treat routinely with folic acid, as well as iron, all cases of anaemia with a haemoglobin of less than 10 g/dl discovered after 28 weeks' gestation.

N.B. This condition is quite distinct from Addisonian pernicious anaemia and it is important to differentiate between them, as folic acid would be bad treatment for the latter. Suspect Addisonian pernicious anaemia in cases of moderately severe or severe anaemia in an older age group, whose anaemia is not known definitely to have occurred in the pregnancy under review. *Investigate* by testing for free stomach acid: if achlorhydric estimate the blood B_{12}.

4. *Sickle-cell Anaemia*—occurs in black ethnic types.

a. Basis. The haemoglobin Hb S/S replaces the more usual Hb A/A.

Carrier state—S/A—about 10% in black people in this country.

Sickle-cell disease—S/S—rare.

b. Effect.

S/A: (*a*) Does not produce anaemia but under hypoxia, e.g. anaesthesia, cells may 'sickle' and disrupt: the resulting crisis produces bone and muscle pains. (*b*) If the husband, too, is S/A there is 1 in 4 chance that a baby would be S/S.

S/S produces: (*a*) Anaemia, e.g. 7–9 g/dl. (*b*) Prematurity, abortion and stillbirth up to a fetal loss of 32%.

c. Detection. (*a*) Sickledex testing at first visit to clinic. (*b*) If positive—electrophoresis on wife and husband to confirm. (*c*) The fetal sickle-cell status can be ascertained by studying fetal blood obtained by: (i) Fetoscopy with aspiration from a placental vessel, or (ii) Placental aspiration, if the parents are prepared to accept termination of pregnancy if the fetus is S/S.

d. Management. (*a*) S/A—special care with oxygenation during anaesthesia. (*b*) S/S—(i) Folic acid supplement. (ii) Blood transfusion (single or exchange) to mother.

(*c*) Consideration of termination of pregnancy if the fetus is established as being S/S.
(*d*) Genetic counselling for the future where both parents are S/A.

5. *Thalassaemia*—occurs mainly in races of Mediterranean origin but also from Middle and Far East.

a. Basis. A variety of disorders of globin, chain production forming haemoglobins of poor oxygen-carrying propensities.

b. Effect. (*a*) (i) *Thalassaemia* trait (heterozygous): May produce mild anaemia (thalassaemia minor) which is iron-refractory. (ii) If both parents have the trait the baby may have thalassaemia major. (*b*) *Thalassaemia major* (homozygous): usually produces severe anaemia. If the fetus has the condition it may produce hydrops fetalis and fetal death.

It is very rare to find a woman with thalassaemia major pregnant.

c. Detection. (*a*) A parent can have a haematological examination to show if he or she carries the trait. Such tests would be done on those of appropriate racial type: (i) Showing *iron-refractory anaemia.* (ii) Perhaps as a *routine* if facilities permit. (*b*) The *fetus* can be examined for the homozygous state by taking fetal blood by fetoscopy or placental aspiration if the parents are prepared to accept termination if the result is positive.

d. Management. (*a*) *Thalassaemia Minor*—folic acid supplements. (*b*) *Thalassaemia Major*—repeated blood transfusions will be required. (*c*) *Fetus with homozygous disease*—termination of pregnancy can be offered.

Diabetes and other Glycosuria

Reducing substances in the urine are nearly always glucose, except near term where lactose is more common due to the increased breast activity.

1. *Alimentary Glycosuria.* There is a rapid rise of the blood sugar level above the renal threshold shortly after a meal (this is due to rapid absorption or to slow storage). The level returns to normal quickly and the fasting blood sugar estimation, too, is normal. This occurs commonly in the first 4 months of pregnancy and is harmless.

2. *Renal Glycosuria.* In this the renal threshold for sugar is low so that a normal blood sugar level leads to excretion of sugar. It has no significance in pregnancy or otherwise.

3. *Diabetes Mellitus*

a. Diagnosis—see under Technique of Antenatal Care, p. 70.

b. Obstetric History (*a*) Large babies. (*b*) Unexplained fetal death in utero and/or neonatal deaths.

Such history may precede the onset of clinical diabetes by 5 or 10 years.

Perhaps the large babies may be produced by excess output of growth hormone from the pituitary gland which may also be producing excess diabetogenic hormone.

c. Severity of Diabetes. May vary from 'gestational diabetes' i.e. glucose intolerance which occurs only when she is pregnant, to severe insulin-dependent diabetes.

d. Fertility. Not affected in a treated case.

e. Maternal Effects. (*a*) Pre-eclampsia—25% of cases compared with 5% in non-diabetics. (*b*) Infection—especially urinary tract infection. (*c*) Lactation often poor; try nevertheless, it is not invariable. (*d*) Monilial vaginitis.

f. Fetal Effects (a perinatal mortality of 8% or less should be aimed at). (*a*) *Abortion and fetal death in utero* after 28 weeks—cause unknown as a rule. (*b*) *Neonatal death:* (1) mainly from *respiratory distress syndrome.* In the normal fetus surfactant is formed in the fetal lung by 35 weeks: in the diabetic it may be delayed until 38 weeks. This will be mirrored in a delayed 'lecithin surge' in the lecithin/sphingomyelin ratio. It may be that the delayed 'lecithin surge' will not occur if the maternal blood sugar is immaculately controlled. (2) *Hypoglycaemia* may occur and need treatment. (*c*) *Large babies* (at 36 weeks' gestation the baby may be as large as at full-term). This may increase the risks to the baby by difficulties at delivery. The increased size has been attributed to high maternal blood sugars but even with near perfect control large babies can still occur: perhaps growth hormone is a factor. (*d*) *Polyhydramnios*—cause unknown. (*e*) *Fetal abnormality*—a small increased incidence.

g. *Effect of Pregnancy on Diabetes*
The disease is more difficult to stabilize and the danger of coma is increased: a higher dose of insulin may be needed and a b.d. or t.d.s. dosage of a short-acting insulin may have to replace a single daily dose of a longer-acting one. *Urine testing* is quite unreliable in pregnancy because of the lowered renal threshold.

h. *Management of Pregnancy*
Careful and painstaking control of the blood sugar level to as near-normal level as possible. This may require long periods of treatment in hospital and in any case:
(*a*) Early in pregnancy for re-stabilization. (*b*) Frequent one day admissions for 'blood sugar profiles', i.e. frequent observation of the blood sugar throughout the day. (*c*) Readmission between 32 and 36 weeks (according to severity) until delivered.

i. *Management of Delivery*
Timing. Usually at 37–38 weeks but certain factors may indicate earlier delivery: (*a*) Rapidly increasing polyhydramnios. (*b*) Rapidly increasing size of the fetal head as determined by ultrasonography. (*c*) Failure of diabetic control. (*d*) Development of pre-eclampsia. (*e*) Intra-uterine death before 38 weeks in a previous pregnancy.

Delay delivery if possible until the lecithin/sphingomyelin ratio is 2:1 or greater, preferably even 3:1 (*vide supra*).
Method. (1) Usually by *surgical induction of labour,* for Caesarean section does not per se

improve the prognosis for the baby; (2) *Caesarean section* if vaginal delivery is delayed or difficult to achieve.

j. Management of the Baby

These babies behave and need managing like premature infants (which indeed they are), despite the fact that they may weigh as much as full-term babies. Special problems are (*a*) Respiratory distress syndrome; (*b*) Hypoglycaemia; (*c*) Hypocalcaemia.

Cardiac Disease

1. *Danger of Mitral Stenosis Associated with Pregnancy*

Mitral stenosis is the commonest lesion. Death may occur from pulmonary oedema (an unusual event in mitral stenosis in the non-pregnant). This is often precipitated by a cough or cold even in cases which were initially well compensated.

2. *Grading of Heart Disease in Pregnancy*

Based on exercise tolerance before onset of pregnancy.

Grade I.   Clinical evidence of a heart lesion but no diminution of exercise tolerance.

Grade II.   Moderate diminution of exercise tolerance.

Grade III. Severe diminution of exercise tolerance not amounting to Grade IV.

Grade IV.   i. Failure past or present, or
             ii. Moist sounds at the lung bases, or
            iii. Auricular fibrillation, or
             iv. Cyanosis in congenital conditions.

3. *Bearing of the Grading on Reproduction*

a. Maternal Mortality: Grade I   0·5%
                          Grade IV 15%

b. Size of Family:

i. There is no evidence, once the admittedly increased risk of pregnancy and labour is past, that the heart suffers permanent damage as a result of childbearing, but the strain of looking after children may cause deterioration.

ii. As a guide one may suggest the following family limitations:

Grade I. A family of two is enough to look after.

Grade IV. This patient runs a considerable risk in childbearing and in general should be advised against it.

Grade II and *III* are considered on their merits after having one child.

4. *Management in Pregnancy*

a. Regular attendance is vital and all cases should be supervised by an obstetrician and a cardiologist working in consultation.

b. The patient should be seen by a *cardiologist* well before the 12th week, if possible, as *termination of pregnancy* is seldom indicated on purely medical grounds after this time. *Valvotomy,* too, has to be considered in suitable cases during pregnancy, where medical measures alone are not likely to be enough.

c. Plans for the pregnancy and afterwards should be made as early as possible in pregnancy, e.g. time when admission to hospital is likely to be required, arrangements for sterilization (including the legal formalities where this is recommended), contraceptive advice, etc.

d. Rest will be required in varying amounts during pregnancy and the appropriate arrangements should be made.

i. Give the patient detailed instruction about how much to rest at home, e.g. two hours lying down in the afternoon and retire to bed at 8 o'clock.

ii. Organize the home so that rest is possible, e.g.:

Home help.

Help from relatives and friends.

Arrange for the children to be cared for by others.

iii. Admission to hospital will be required according to the severity of the lesion. (*a*) All cases are admitted a week or two before confinement. (*b*) Severe cases will be admitted as required and the worst ones may spend most of pregnancy in hospital.

e. Anaemia should be diagnosed and treatment begun as early as possible.

f. Respiratory tract infections, even minor coughs and colds, are dangerous. The patient should be advised to retire to bed and to notify her own doctor.

g. Decompensation is treated fully by medical means (rest, digitalis, etc.) before any thought is given to the further management of the pregnancy itself.

5. *Management in Labour*

a. Antibiotic cover is often recommended at the onset of labour to prevent subacute bacterial endocarditis, e.g. streptomycin and penicillin.

b. A very careful watch must be kept on the maternal condition, especially the pulse rate, and any change reported at once.

c. Notify the obstetrician when the second stage begins as this is often shortened by forceps delivery, preferably under local anaesthesia.

N.B. Cardiac cases usually have exceptionally easy normal deliveries and take labour well. The more severe the case, the more important it is to get a vaginal delivery. Elective abdominal delivery is reserved for those few cases where considerable difficulty is anticipated in vaginal delivery.

Urinary Tract Infection

1. *Cause*

This infection is common in pregnancy due to urinary stasis produced by: (*a*) Progesterone relaxing smooth muscle. (*b*) Back-pressure from the gravid uterus.

2. *Symptoms*

a. Cystitis: (i) Frequency (particularly nocturnal). (ii) Scalding.

b. Pyelitis: (i) Pain over one or both loins. (ii) Symptoms of cystitis (as above). (iii) Malaise (if severe infection).

3. *Signs*
a. Tenderness over the affected kidney in pyelitis.
b. Pyrexia in severe infections.
c. Pus cells are seen in a catheter specimen of urine under the microscope.
4. *Management*
a. A *mid-stream specimen* of urine must be sent to the laboratory for culture *before* starting antibiotics.
b. *Antibiotic treatment.* (i) Amoxycillin 250 mg t.d.s. for 5–7 days is a reasonable choice for 'blind' treatment. (ii) Failure to respond will call for a change of antibiotic dictated by the sensitivity report.
c. *Recurrent infections or relapse.* (i) Investigate more fully, e.g. intravenous pyelogram, serum creatinine, etc. (ii) Give a longer course of an appropriate antibiotic. (iii) Prophylaxis, e.g. Nitrofurantoin 50 mg *nocte,* if continual recurrence.
d. *Asymptomatic bacteriuria.* (i) *Detection*— routine testing by dip-stick. (ii) *Danger*—in pregnancy 50% will develop clinical infection. (iii) *Treatment*—*appropriate antibiotic.*

Glomerulonephritis
1. *Cardinal Signs*
a. Proteinuria.
b. Hypertension.
Oedema and haematuria may also be present.
2. *Clinical Presentation*
a. *Acute Nephritis* is very rare in pregnancy and is purely coincidental.
b. *Chronic Glomerulonephritis:* (i) Proteinuria —variable in amount, seldom severe.
(ii) Hypertension—moderate to severe.
c. *Nephrotic Syndrome* (i) Proteinuria— marked. (ii) Oedema—severe.
(iii) Hypertension—variable; may be absent.
3. *Diagnosis from Pre-eclampsia*
In the *first half of pregnancy* it is easy but as pregnancy proceeds *towards term* it becomes difficult or impossible without renal biopsy.

After *delivery* pre-eclampsia clears up within days or weeks—rarely months: if proteinuria and hypertension persist, investigation is required.

4. *Dangers*

a. Maternal (i) Deterioration of renal function. (ii) Increased severity of hypertension in pregnancy and afterwards.

b. Fetal (i) Fetal death. (ii) Low birth weight. (iii) Accidental haemorrhage.

5. *Prognosis*

a. Mild cases will go through pregnancy without problems or deterioration of condition.

b. Severe cases, e.g. with (i) Serum creatinine in excess of 200 μmol/l, (ii) Blood pressure of greater than 160/90 mmHg, have increased risks both in pregnancy and afterwards.

6. *Management*

a. Close monitoring of fetal and maternal condition throughout.

b. Delivery of baby prematurely, taking all factors into account.

Syphilis

1. *Effect on Baby*

a. Late abortion (not under 24 weeks).

b. Stillbirth.

c. Congenital syphilitic live birth; signs may: (i) Be apparent at birth, or (ii) Appear while under observation in hospital, or (iii) Be delayed up to age of adolescence.

N.B. Placenta looks large, pale and greasy. Exceeds quarter the weight of the baby (normal is one-sixth).

2. *Treatment*

a. In Pregnancy: The mother should be seen by a venereologist and penicillin will usually be ordered in each pregnancy to ensure an unaffected baby.

b. After Delivery: (i) The baby is observed closely and a watch kept for stigmata (including X-ray of long bones). (ii) The baby will be treated with penicillin unless the paediatrician is confident that it is unaffected.

Pulmonary Tuberculosis

1. *Effect of Pregnancy on the Disease*
Only active infection is adversely affected by pregnancy and termination of pregnancy is almost never indicated on purely medical grounds.

2. *Management*
a. Treat the patient in the same way that would be indicated were she not pregnant, though, as a rule, major chest surgery would be delayed until after pregnancy.

b. Deliver the patient where both an obstetrician and a chest physician are available.

c. If instrumental delivery is required it is best performed under local anaesthesia.

d. Inoculate the baby with BCG vaccine, isolating it for 6 weeks if the maternal disease is active.

e. Breast-feeding is contra-indicated if the disease is active; in other cases, opinion is divided.

Thyrotoxicosis

1. *Effect on Pregnancy*
No marked effect.

2. *Effect of Pregnancy on the Disease*
May make it worse but usually does not affect it.

3. *Management*
As in the non-pregnant (including operation if indicated), but carbimazole (Neo-Mercazole) must be used with caution as it gives the baby a goitre and neonatal hypothyroidism.

Rubella

Effect on Pregnancy
The main effects are only produced by rubella in the first 12 weeks of pregnancy, and to a minor extent between 12 and 16 weeks. No effects can be demonstrated after that time (*see* p. 135).

Thrombo-embolism

1. *Incidence of Maternal Death* from the *Confidential Report into Maternal Death in England and Wales 1976–1978.*

Deaths from pulmonary embolism	45
Antenatal deaths	14
Postpartum deaths	31

N.B. Antenatal cases represent nearly one-third of the total.

Premonitory symptoms and signs were present in 6 of the 14 antenatal deaths e.g. chest pain, superficial and deep thrombosis in the leg. Such cases need urgent attention (*see below*).

2. *Clinical Aspects*

See Puerperal Thrombo-embolic Phenomena, p. 213.

3. *Management in Pregnancy*

a. Immediate treatment of all thrombo-embolism

Heparin by: (i) Intermittent i.v. route (*see* p. 217) or (ii) Intravenous infusion—40000 units in 24 hours.

Continue for up to 7 days, then follow prophylactic regime (*see below*).

b. Prophylaxis

Indications (i) History of previous thrombo-embolism, whether in pregnancy or not. (ii) Follow up after full heparinization. (iii) In cases of doubtful diagnosis or not considered severe enough for full heparinization.

Method (i) *Heparin calcium* 5000 units bd self administered. Supplied as Calciparine in disposable syringes. (ii) *Warfarin. Dangers in pregnancy*—may affect the fetus, e.g. chondrodysplasia punctata, nasal hypoplasia, small-for-dates, brachydactylia. All these have been reported in the first 12 weeks of pregnancy but the incidence is not high. *Use* after 14 weeks' gestation if the patient cannot manage the self-administered heparin.

Cease prophylaxis at 38 weeks' gestation and induce labour. Commence Warfarin 48 hours after delivery and continue until 6 weeks postpartum.

Detect Certain Conditions which Arise in Pregnancy

The first three conditions are commonly listed together under the general title of 'toxaemias'. This is a bad term as there is no evidence of a 'toxin' and moreover it suggests an association between some of the conditions which in fact does not exist.

The most important conditions are:

Pre-eclampsia and Eclampsia, q.v.

Antepartum Haemorrhage, q.v.

Hyperemesis Gravidarum, q.v.

Postmaturity

1. *The Problem.* There is evidence that when a pregnancy exceeds 42 weeks there is an increased incidence of stillbirth due to placental insufficiency produced by the development of the fetus outstripping the ability of the placenta to supply it. (Even at full term the baby is in a precarious situation with regard to oxygenation, as demonstrated by its high haemoglobin and red-cell count values; cf. mountaineers acclimatized at high altitudes.)

2. *Factors to Consider in Diagnosing Postmaturity*

a. The certainty of the last menstrual period date.

b. The regularity and length of the menstrual cycle.

c. Confirmation of the period of gestation earlier in pregnancy: (1) Height of fundus up to 24 weeks (error up to $\pm$ 4 weeks). (2) Ultrasound assessment before 30 weeks and preferably 20 weeks (error up to $\pm$ 2 weeks). *N.B.* If ultrasound dating is not available and any of the other factors are in doubt it is impossible to diagnose postmaturity with confidence.

3. *Management*

If there is reasonable confidence in the expected date of confinement most obstetricians advocate surgical induction of labour when the baby is 2 weeks overdue. A minority of obstetricians may induce earlier.

Surgical induction of labour at full term should be safe and easy, but if there are factors decreasing the safety or ease of the manoeuvre then it is better to wait (for the risks of postmaturity to the fetus are not great), or to consider Caesarean section if the problem delaying action is not likely to resolve itself, e.g. disproportion, unstable lie, etc.

Fetal Growth Retardation ('Small-for-dates' Baby)

1. *Definition*

Sometimes the fetus seems clinically to be small for the period of gestation and it fails to grow adequately. Such babies are not only small and dysmature at birth but may die in utero. It is presumed to be due to placental insufficiency. This may be associated with pre-eclampsia, essential hypertension and nephritis, but it may occur without any such association. It may rarely be observed in successive pregnancies perhaps leading to fetal death in utero at about 36 weeks.

2. *Diagnosis*

a. Suspect. i. When the baby seems to be unusually small for the period of gestation. *N.B.* (1) Clinical assessment of fetal size is notoriously inaccurate. (2) The calculated period of gestation may be in error.

ii. If an ultrasound examination has been performed routinely or for some other reason and the fetal measurements are smaller than expected.

b. Confirmation

i. *Ultrasonography*

Method. Serial measurements: (1) Biparietal diameter. (2) Abdominal circumference (more closely related to weight than head measurements). (3) Circumference of the head (if head/abdomen ratio is required).

Interpretation. Growth retardation is confirmed if: (1) *Biparietal diameters* are below what would be expected when related to that attained with an *ultrasound examination made in early pregnancy*. (2) *Successive observations on biparietal diameter* or *abdominal circumference* fall away from the standard graph. (3) Relatively greater fall away of abdominal circumference compared with the head circumference (asymmetrical growth retardation).

N.B. If head and abdominal circumference fall equally (symmetrical growth retardation), it suggests innate growth failure, or even a congenital abnormality causing poor growth, rather than placental insufficiency.

ii. *Oestriol Secretion of Placenta*

Measured by: (1) *Oestriol-creatinine index* on an early morning specimen of urine (quick result, easy to take and gives a reliable prediction). (2) *Serum oestriol* (quick result and easy to take but may be vitiated by fluid intake). (3) *Urinary oestriol* on a 24-hour specimen. This is the least satisfactory as: (*a*) the container is cumbersome to carry around; (*b*) it loses a day—that of collection; (*c*) collection is liable to be inaccurate and therefore unreliable. However, if properly performed, i.e. under supervision, may give the most reliable prediction.

iii. *Fetal Cardiotocography*

Method. A 20–30 minute run on the machine. *Interpretation.* (1) *A flat trace* viz. with little fetal reactivity, e.g. to contractions—an adverse sign. (2) *Marked 'dips'*—a serious warning.

3. *Management*

Deliver the baby, weighing the risks of prematurity against those of remaining in utero.

N.B. In most cases when a 'small-for-dates' baby is suspected, events prove either that the clinical assessment was in error or the dates were misleading. To deliver such a baby prematurely which was not at risk in utero could be disastrous. True growth retardation is not common.

ANTENATAL DIAGNOSIS OF FETAL ABNORMALITIES

Classification of Fetal Disorders

Chromosomal Abnormalities

Notably *trisomy 21* (Down's syndrome) (other abnormalities occur but are numerically less important).

Types of chromosomal defect in trisomy 21:

i. Non-disjunction (95% of cases of Down's syndrome). Age related:

Age	Incidence
15–19	1 : 2300
20–24	1 : 1600
25–29	1 : 1200
30–34	1 : 880
35–39	1 : 290
40–44	1 : 100
45–49	1 : 50

ii. Translocation (5% of cases of Down's syndrome) (*a*) Occurs as a rule in younger women; (*b*) Chromosomal studies in the parents will reveal an abnormality; (*c*) Risk of a further affected child if the translocation is carried by the father—2–3%; the mother—about 10%.

Metabolic Disorders

Methods of inheritance

i. Autosomal recessive, or

ii. X-linked recessive.

Diseases concerned (caused by enzyme deficiencies)

i. CONDITIONS DIAGNOSABLE AT PRESENT IN THE MID-TRIMESTER OF PREGNANCY (Number about 70 but the field is growing rapidly). They are all rare—some very rare. Examples:

(*a*) Tay–Sachs disease: (i) Mainly in Ashkenazi Jews, 1 in 27 of whom are said to be carriers, identified by estimating serum hexosaminidase A activity. (ii) Caused by

deficiency of hexosaminidase A activity and
an affected fetus can be detected by
amniocentesis.

(*b*) Gaucher's disease.

(*c*) Galactosaemia.

(*d*) Congenital adrenal hyperplasia.

ii. IMPORTANT METABOLIC CONDITIONS FOR
WHICH ANTENATAL DIAGNOSIS IN THE 2ND
TRIMESTER IS NOT AVAILABLE AT PRESENT

(*a*) Phenylketonuria.

(*b*) Hypothyroidism.

iii. X-LINKED RECESSIVE CONDITIONS
(The mother is a carrier and it affects male
children).

Examples:

(*a*) Haemophilia—antenatal diagnosis is
possible by examining fetal blood.

(*b*) Duchenne's muscular dystrophy—not yet
diagnosable in utero.

Management:

(*a*) Termination of pregnancy with a male
fetus will prevent the birth of affected children
but will be achieved at the cost of destroying
some unaffected male fetuses as only 50% are
affected.

(*b*) With antenatal diagnosis by fetal blood
sampling, selective termination of pregnancy in
only affected male fetuses can be offered.

Neural Tube Defects (NTD)

a. Spina Bifida and Anencephaly

RISK OF RECURRENCE:

(*a*) one previous incident 1/20.

(*b*) two previous incidents 1/8.

DETECTION:

(i) *Ultrasonography.*

PERIOD OF GESTATION: (*a*) *Anencephaly* from
14–15 weeks. (*b*) *Spina bifida* between 14
and 18 weeks is the best time. Repeat examinations are necessary to exclude spina bifida
with reasonable confidence in high risk cases.

SELECTION OF CASES: (*a*) *Previous incident* of
NTD. (*b*) *Family history* of NTD. (*c*) *Raised
serum α-fetoprotein on routine screening:* (1)

To confirm the presence or absence of NTD.
(2) To reassess the period of gestation as an
error in the calculation of this might have
given rise to the reported raised α-fetoprotein
level as this is very critically related to the
period of gestation. (*d*) *Routine ultrasound
screening at 14–18 weeks* where facilities
permit. It is likely that this will eventually
replace routine screening by maternal serum
α-fetoprotein level.

(ii) MATERNAL SERUM α-FETOPROTEIN LEVEL.
(*a*) The level is raised between 16 and 18
weeks in 88% of anencephalics and in 79% of
spina bifida cases: thus there is a significant
number of false negatives and closed spina
bifida cases are not picked up (about 10%).
(*b*) There is a significant number of false
positives. Some of these are due to
overestimation of the period of gestation and
ultrasound confirmation of this is required:
even so, unexplained raised levels occur. (*c*) If
the level is raised: (1) Repeat the estimation.
(2) If still raised perform ultrasonography to
confirm dates—new date may make the
fetoprotein level normal—and prove, or
disprove, the presence of NTD. (3) If
α-fetoprotein still considered raised and
NTD not seen, perform amniocentesis for
α-fetoprotein estimation.

(iii) AMNIOTIC α-FETOPROTEIN LEVEL.
(*a*) The period of gestation materially affects
the interpretation of the result. Therefore
ultrasound confirmation is vital. (*b*) If there is
an *open spina bifida or anencephaly* a positive
result is almost always obtained. Closed *spina
bifida* gives a negative result. (*c*) *False
positives* occur in: (1) specimens contaminated
by blood; (2) 0·15% of cases without
explanation. (*d*) *Use* (1) to confirm doubtful
ultrasound results; (2) with raised serum
α-fetoprotein and a negative ultrasound report.

b. *Hydrocephaly*
METHOD OF DIAGNOSIS: by ultrasound
(i) head well outside normal size for period of

gestation; (ii) ventricles enlarged; (iii) may be an associated spina bifida.
PERIOD OF GESTATION: usually investigated in third trimester. May be picked up in the middle trimester.

Some other Anatomical Abnormalities Diagnosable by Ultrasound

i. Fetal ascites—usually associated with serious abnormalities of the fetus. May give difficulty at delivery.

ii. Exomphalos.

iii. Duodenal atresia—associated with polyhydramnios.

iv. Renal agenesis—associated with oligohydramnios.

v. Achondroplasia—difficult to identify (80% are new mutations).

Haemoglobinopathies (*see above*).
Sickle-cell anaemia and thalassaemia.

Other Genetically Determined Conditions for which at Present no Method of Diagnosis in Utero Exists

AUTOSOMAL DOMINANTS
(1 : 2 chance of a child being affected if one parent has the condition).

i. *Achondroplasia (can sometimes be picked up by ultrasound).*

ii. *Huntington's chorea* (condition often not apparent in parent until after childbearing is over, but recent discoveries based on DNA technique, may make it possible to identify those who can pass on the disease).

N.B. Children with these conditions may be new mutations.

AUTOSOMAL RECESSIVE
(1 : 4 chance of an affected child if both parents are carriers).

Cystic fibrosis (no test exists at present to identify carriers, so the situation is not apparent until after the first affected child is born).

Clinical Situation leading to Investigation and Antenatal Diagnosis

Routine Screening

CRITERIA TO MAKE IT COST EFFECTIVE IN TERMS OF TIME AND MONEY
a. The condition should be sufficiently frequent in the community being studied. *b*. The screening tests on the parents (if applicable) and on the fetus should be: (i) reliable, and (ii) reasonably quick and inexpensive, and (iii) safe.
Examples:
(*a*) The whole community. Neural tube defects—by ultrasound or maternal serum α-fetoprotein. (*b*) Selected groups.

Condition	Group	Parents	Fetus
Sickle-cell anaemia	Black races	Sickledex and electrophoresis	Fetal blood study
Tay–Sachs disease	Ashkenazi Jews	Parental serum	Amniocentesis

Birth of an Affected Child

(Studies are worth pursuing if the parents will accept termination of pregnancy if offered and where applicable).
Examples:

Condition(s)	Parents	Future Pregnancy
Trisomy 21	Chromosome studies	Amniocentesis in future
Metabolic disorders	Serum studies	Amniocentesis in future
Haemophilia		Fetal blood study
Duchenne's muscular dystrophy		Amniocentesis. Offer termination if male
Neural tube defects		i. Ultrasound ii. Amniocentesis

Family History
Examples: (i) Haemophilia; (ii) Duchenne's muscular dystrophy (but one-third of cases are new mutations).

Age of Mother
Trisomy 21.

Routine Obstetrical Antenatal Examinations

Poly-hydramnios	– spina bifida; anencephaly	– ultrasound or X-ray
Oligo-hydramnios	– renal agenesis	– ultrasound
Large head and/or disproportion	– hydrocephaly	– ultrasound or X-ray
Small head	– anencephaly or micro-cephaly	– ultrasound or X-ray

Objects of Parental Investigation and Antenatal Diagnosis

a. Termination of pregnancy if the parents wish this where: (i) The fetus certainly, or almost certainly, has a serious disorder; (ii) There is a high risk of such a disorder, e.g. X-linked recessive conditions (50% risk if male): Cystic fibrosis (25% risk).
b. Planning obstetric management.
(i) Induction of premature labour with abnormalities incompatible with life (e.g. *anencephaly),* (ii) Craniotomy with *hydrocephaly* unless very borderline in size, (iii) Paracentesis with *gross fetal ascites.*
c. Making preparations for treatment of the baby as soon as possible. This is important in certain types of case, e.g. congenital adrenal hypoplasia; galactosaemia.
d. Genetic counselling with a view to the future. Most centres have access to a consultative clinic.

Methods of Antenatal Diagnosis Available

Parents

(i) *Chromosome analysis* after birth of a child with trisomy 21 or other chromosomal abnormality. (ii) *Blood examination* in *sickle-cell disease* and *thalassaemia* by electrophoresis. (iii) *Maternal serum α-fetoprotein* for open neural tube defects. An exact knowledge of the period of gestation is critical and it is advisable for this to be confirmed by ultrasonography.

Fetus in utero

a. Ultrasonography for (i) neural tube defects (*see above*); (ii) growth retardation (*see above*); (iii) fetal ascites; (iv) exomphalos; (v) duodenal atresia; (vi) renal agenesis; (vii) achondroplasia; (viii) period of gestation.

b. Amniocentesis

FEASIBLE from 16 weeks onwards.

RISK OF INDUCED ABORTION—about 0·5%.

METHODS

(i) CELL-FREE AMNIOTIC FLUID for:

(1) *Neural tube defects* (α-feto-protein) where ultrasonography is doubtful or *serum α-fetoprotein* is raised and ultrasonography is not available.

(2) *Some metabolic disorders* e.g. Tay–Sachs disease (hexosaminidase A) and adrenal hyperplasia (17-ketosteroids).

(3) Also used late in pregnancy to assess: the fetal condition in erythroblastosis (bilirubin) and fetal pulmonary maturity by lecithin/sphingomyelin ratio.

(ii) UNCULTIVATED FREE CELLS IN AMNIOTIC FLUID (mainly from amnion): in some metabolic disorders—probably unreliable.

(iii) CULTIVATED FREE CELLS IN AMNIOTIC FLUID (requires 3 weeks) for: (1) Chromosome abnormality, e.g. trisomy 21. (2) X-linked conditions to establish sex of fetus. (3) Metabolic disorders, e.g. Tay–Sachs disease.

c. Examination of Fetal Blood

METHODS (i) Fetoscopy. (ii) Placental aspiration.

INDICATIONS. To diagnose and offer termination of pregnancy in: (i) Sickle-cell disease if fetus is S/S (ii) Thalassaemia if fetus has the major form. (In (i) and (ii) both parents will be heterozygous.) (iii) Haemophilia if it is a male child to see if it is affected. (iv) Some metabolic disorders.

d. Transcervical or Transabdominal Biopsy of Chorion

(at the time of writing these techniques are only in the experimental phase).

METHOD. Aspiration of chorionic material in early pregnancy.

ADVANTAGE. Material can be evaluated while termination of pregnancy by the vaginal route is still safe, e.g. in diagnosis of trisomy 21.

ANTICIPATION OF DIFFICULTIES IN LABOUR

1. Contracted pelvis.
2. Abnormal presentation, particularly breech and transverse lie.
3. Polyhydramnios.
4. Multiple pregnancy.
5. Abnormal fetus, e.g. hydrocephaly, fetal ascites, etc.

HYGIENE OF PREGNANCY

Work, Exercise and Recreation.
In moderation, unless specially contra-indicated.
Low back pain, due to the altered weight-bearing attitude in late pregnancy, is common. Rest is required. More serious problems are:
a. Disc lesions with *sciatic pain.*
b. Pelvic osteoarthropathy. This is due to softening of the ligaments of the sacro-iliac joints in the symphysis pubis producing pain over those joints which can be disabling. Actual movement of one pubic bone on the

other can be demonstrated when standing first on one foot and then on the other.

The condition clears up as a rule within weeks of delivery.

It is rare.

Smoking leads to a reduction in average birth weight by about 500 g. Many women find a loss of the desire to smoke in pregnancy: encourage this to be permanent.

Dress. Avoid constriction of abdomen, breasts and thighs, especially in late pregnancy. Provide elastic stockings for varicose veins which are likely to produce symptoms.

Sleep. Treat insomnia by general measures such as reassurance, hot drinks at nights, etc. A tendency to rely on hypnotic drugs should be avoided.

Coitus. Unwise to forbid altogether. Advise against it: (*a*) At the time when the third missed period would have been due. (*b*) In the last month of pregnancy.

Breasts
1. *General Discomfort*
a. Early pregnancy—avoid pressure but no special treatment required.
b. Late pregnancy—support with suitable binder as the ordinary brassière compresses the nipples too much.
2. *Nipples.* Keep them supple by use of lanoline. Alcohol and scrubbing are to be deprecated. It is doubtful whether the use of Waller nipple shells improves the quality of the nipple for breast-feeding: poor nipples tend to improve in pregnancy without special treatment (Hytten F. E. (1954) Br. Med. J. 2, 1451).

Alimentary Tract
1. *Teeth.* Seek attention as early as possible in pregnancy: do not wait until after delivery.
2. *Nausea and Sickness*
a. Reassure that as a rule it passes off by about the 16th week.

b. Dietetic advice—'little and often'; eat food dry, drinking between meals.

3. *Heartburn.* Alkalis, e.g. Aluminium Hydroxide Mixture (gel.) 5–15 ml, prn. If fails: Mucaine 5–10 ml, tds, ac and at bedtime.

4. *Constipation*

a. (i) Natural remedies: exercise, adequate fluids, 'roughage' (fruit, green vegetables, wholemeal bread, miller's bran one tablespoonful tds sprinkled on food, etc.). (ii) Attempt to cultivate a regular habit for bowel action: dyschezia, or chronic absence of the desire to defaecate because the urge has been ignored, is common in pregnancy.

b. Purgatives: Senokot—preferably not more than once per week.

c. Bulk-increasers, e.g. Isogel 2 teaspoonfuls bd ex aqua pc, or Normacol Special 2 teaspoonfuls bd pc.

5. *Haemorrhoids*

a. Cure constipation.

b. Suppos. Bism. Subgall.

c. If they stay persistently prolapsed, seek early medical advice.

Diet (in pregnancy and lactation)

a. Theoretical daily needs (based on recommendations of the Health Committee of the League of Nations):

Calories	2700
Protein	100 g
Fat	100 g
Carbohydrate	300 g
Salts: Calcium	1·5 g
Iron	20 mg
Vitamins: A	9000 IU
B complex	1 mg
C (ascorbic acid)	75 mg
D (calciferol)	700 IU

b. General guide to diet (Mellanby):

Milk	Two pints per day
Green vegetables	Once or twice per day
Eggs	Once or twice per day

Fresh fruit	Daily
Fish	Twice per week
Liver	Once per week
Meat	Daily, except when fish or liver is eaten

Supplements
| Ferrous sulphate | 200 mg daily |
| Folic acid | 5 mg daily |

Many give these supplements but some only treat if the haemoglobin level demands it (*see under* 'Anaemia', p. 42).

N.B. Do not become, or turn your patient into, a dietetic crank.

TECHNIQUE OF ANTENATAL CARE

Frequency of Attendance

1. First attendance should be within the first 12 weeks.
2. Thence monthly till 28 weeks.
3. Thence at fortnightly intervals until 36 weeks.
4. Thence weekly until delivered.
N.B. Keep a flexible attitude towards return visits. Special cases may need more frequent attendance, e.g.:
a. Cases of anaemia need supervision to ensure that they are taking their therapy and to follow progress.
b. Patients with hypertension, finger oedema, or excessive weight gain should be seen frequently, occasionally at even less than weekly intervals.
c. Where there is a history of previous severe and early pre-eclampsia, or of accidental haemorrhage, a weekly visit for blood pressure reading, from the 24th week, is indicated.

First Visit

History
a. Age and age at marriage.
b. Married or single.
c. Previous medical and surgical history.
d. Menstrual history (particularly the date of the last period and the length and regularity of the cycle).

e. Obstetrical history.

f. History of present pregnancy, e.g. nausea and vomiting, frequency of, or pain during micturition, vaginal discharge, vulval irritation, vaginal bleeding, abdominal pain, constipation, dyspnoea, etc.

Investigations

1. *Blood*

a. Haemoglobin estimation—2 ml with anticoagulant.

b. Blood grouping (ABO and Rh) with screening test for atypical antibodies.

c. VDRL test for syphilis.

d. Rubella antibody test for immunity (this is not necessary if a previous test has shown immunity).

e. Serum α-fetoprotein (if considered worthwhile—*see* p. 60).

f. Sickledex test (on black patients)—*see* p. 44).

g. Test for thalassaemia trait (on races of Mediterranean origin and from the Middle and Far East—*see* p. 45).

h. Test for Hepatitis B carriers (HBV; Australia antigen). If positive for HB_sAg, test for HB_eAg.

INDICATIONS

Patients from certain parts of the Far East e.g. Vietnam with a history of: (1) Jaundice. (2) Drug addiction by injection. (3) Excessive promiscuity.

OBJECT

(1) To eliminate the carrier state in babies born of mothers carrying HB_eAg. (2) to prevent late morbidity with cirrhosis or hepatocellular carcinoma.

METHOD

Passive immunization with hepatitis B immune globulin (HBIG) within 48 hours of birth and then monthly for 6 months.

Active immunization of neonates is not at present authorized but may become the practice at a future date.

2. *Ultrasonography*

Not recommended as a routine at the first antenatal visit to confirm period of gestation unless it is already thought to be at least 14 weeks. May be indicated: (i) To demonstrate pregnancy, if necessary. (ii) To show the fetus is active if this be in doubt, especially if there has been bleeding. (iii) Where there is a suspicion of a para-uterine mass.

General Medical Examination by the Doctor

Routine General Examination (*see below*)

Obstetric Examination

a. Breasts and nipples.

b. Abdominal (*see below*)

c. Vaginal examination is useful at the first visit to:

 i. Confirm pregnancy (if less than 12 weeks).

 ii. Detect vaginal discharges.

iii. Diagnose fibroids, ovarian cysts or other tumours in the pelvis.

iv. Measure the diagonal conjugate (not always possible, but useful if home confinement is being planned).

 v. Perform a cervical smear if this has not been done in the previous 3 years.

All Visits

Routine General Examination

1. *Urine for:*

a. Proteinuria. If positive take a mid-stream specimen and test part of it for protein. If still positive send the rest to the laboratory to be examined for urinary infection.

b. Glucose. If positive on 2 occasions arrange a blood-sugar estimation 2 hours after a carbohydrate meal: if this is greater than 6 mmol/l a glucose tolerance test should be done.

Top limits of acceptability: fasting 5 mmol/l; 1 hour 8 mmol/l; 2 hours 6 mmol/l.

c. Ketones. If patient has been vomiting or if sugar is present.

d. Nitrite. If positive, examine a mid-stream specimen for urinary infection.

2. *Weight.* This is not done at all clinics. The patient should be weighed in the same garment and on the same scales at each visit. The scales should be jockey scales or of the beam pattern—spring ones are too inaccurate. A gain of more than 2 kg in any period of 4 weeks may be the first sign of impending pre-eclampsia.

3. *Blood Pressure*

4. *Oedema*

a. Pitting of feet and over tibiae.

b. Ask if wedding ring is getting tighter.

Abdominal Examination

1. *Inspection* (only in third trimester)

a. Lie of fetus.

b. Side on which back lies.

c. Presence and site of fetal movements.

d. Occipitoposterior position. Abdomen concave below the umbilicus, and fetal movements on both sides of midline.

e. Abdominal oedema.

2. Palpation

a. Information to be gained:

Period of gestation to nearest 2 weeks.

Presenting part, its position and its level (only in third trimester).

Number of babies.

Detection of polyhydramnios.

Detection of uterine abnormality, e.g. fibroids, double uterus, etc.

b. Techniques:

Height of Fundus:

12 weeks—just palpable above the pubis.

16 weeks—midway between umbilicus and pubic symphysis.

20 weeks—just below the umbilicus (22 weeks at the umbilicus.)

24 weeks—just above the umbilicus.

28 weeks—at the junction of the lower one-third and upper two-thirds of the distance between the umbilicus and the ensiform cartilage.

32 weeks—at the junction of the lower two-thirds and upper one-third of the distance between the umbilicus and the ensiform cartilage.

36 weeks—at the ensiform cartilage.

40 weeks—as for 32 weeks, but:

The presenting part will be low.

The uterus will be broader and the general size of the baby greater.

N.B. It is assumed that the presenting part enters the pelvis between the 36th and the 40th week. If it should enter earlier, the period of gestation, after the 28th week, may be 4 weeks more than the height of the fundus indicates.

Preliminary Pelvic Palpation: What is the presenting part?

Two-handed technique or deep pelvic palpation (the only method if the presenting part is very deep). One-handed technique or Pawlik's grip (more suitable for the high presenting part).

Fundal Palpation: What is in the fundus?

Two-handed technique.

One-handed technique.

Lateral Palpation: Where lies the back? Is it anterior or posterior in position? Are there any more fetal poles?

Final Pelvic Palpation: What is the level of the presenting part? In the case of a head presenting, is it well flexed?

The head can be described as being:

(1) High and mobile.

(2) At the brim (sitting in the brim but not through).

(3) Engaged (largest diameter is past the brim).

(4) Deeply engaged (the head is almost out of reach).

Auscultation

Examinations at Certain Visits to the Clinic

Repeat Blood Test for Rh Antibodies

1. *Selection of cases*

a. All Rh-negative patients (except in first pregnancy).

b. Patients with a history of neonatal jaundice, unexplained stillbirths and neonatal deaths, etc.

2. *Time of tests*
At 28 weeks' and 34 weeks' gestation.

Haemoglobin Estimation
At least at first visit and 34 weeks but ideally more often if possible, perhaps monthly, and certainly whenever blood is taken for any other purpose.

There should be facilities to make the result available while the patient is at the clinic.

Ultrasonography
Not known to have any adverse affect on fetus.
Uses
a. To *diagnose early pregnancy*—much more effective than hormonal pregnancy tests.
b. To resolve doubts about *viability of the pregnancy,* especially if there has been bleeding. Possible abnormal findings:
(i) Blighted ovum i.e. sac but not fetus;
(ii) Fetus but no fetal heart beat seen on real-time scan—from 6 weeks onwards;
(iii) Hydatidiform mole q.v.; (iv) Retained products of conception but no fetus. In all these cases a D and C is required except where a fetus is greater than 12 weeks in size.
c. To establish the *period of gestation* and the *expected date of confinement. Importance*—when delivery of the baby is contemplated either prematurely e.g. with pre-eclampsia, or if postmaturity is suspected. *Optimal period of gestation* for a *routine examination* which is recommended in all cases is between 14 and 20 weeks. This is also a good time, as scanning, to exclude neural tube defects, can be performed at the same time. *Method* by crown–rump length up to 10 weeks; by biparietal from 12 weeks.
d. To detect *fetal abnormality,* especially *neural tube defects* (*see above*), and also
e. To detect *multiple pregnancy.*
f. To confirm the presence of *para-uterine tumours in early pregnancy.*

g. To *locate the placenta:* (i) In suspected placenta praevia, antepartum haemorrhage, a high or unstable presenting part.
N.B. Placenta praevia may be a chance finding when ultrasonography is being performed for some other reason.
(ii) To locate a 'window' before performing amniocentesis.
h. To assess *fetal growth* (*see* p. 56).
Selection of cases: (i) When the fetus seems clinically to be 'small-for-dates'; (ii) Where placental insufficiency is likely, e.g. in pre-eclampsia; (iii) As a routine on all cases, when facilities permit, between 30 and 34 weeks to pick up unsuspected growth retardation.
Methods: The essence of the technique is observing serial readings. Two weeks apart is the least worthwhile interval. Readings should be recorded on a special graph: (i) Biparietal diameter; (ii) Abdominal circumference; (iii) Head circumference/abdominal circumference ratio.
i. *Cord presentation.*

X-radiology
Must be avoided in pregnancy wherever possible, especially in the first trimester.
Uses
a. *Pelvimetry* and to assess cephalopelvic relationship.
b. To confirm fetal death in utero.
c. To diagnose multiple pregnancy.
d. To diagnose *skeletal fetal abnormality.*

Estimation of Cephalopelvic Relationship and Detection of Contracted Pelvis at 36 Weeks
This should be considered in multigravidae as well as in primigravidae. The adequacy of the pelvis cannot be assumed despite the birth of previous babies of a good weight.
Proceed as follows:
1. If the *head is in the pelvis* there will be no disproportion at term. If not, perform

2. *Head Fitting*

a. In horizontal position, or

b. In the semi-sitting position, leaning back on the arms, or

c. Standing up, leaning forward on the arms. If it fails:

3. *a.* Estimate the pelvis by *vaginal examination,* measuring the diagonal conjugate. Subtract 1·5 cm to give an approximation to the internal conjugate, and

b. Attempt a *bi-manual head fitting* by Müller's method and Munro-Kerr's modification of it.

4. *X-ray Pelvimetry* may be resorted to if all the above manoeuvres fail. It is also employed as a routine in cases where breech delivery is contemplated in a primigravid patient and may be necessary in some multigravid breech cases where the pelvic size is in doubt.

N.B. There has been a trend for some years in some quarters to regard this formal assessment of cephalo-pelvic relationship as unnecessary; this tendency is to be deprecated.

4

Vaginal Discharge

There are four main causes of vaginal discharge in the woman of reproductive age, excluding cases where the discharge is secondary to some other condition, e.g. cervical polyp, foreign body, etc. (*see Table* I).

SOME FURTHER POINTS

1. At the first visit to the antenatal clinic, the presence of a discharge should be ascertained by direct questions and examination if necessary. The patient will often fail to volunteer information in response to a more general question.

2. A full investigation for vaginal discharge consists of:

a. A vaginal swab ⎫ Sent to the laboratory
b. A urethral swab ⎬ within half an hour
c. An endocervical ⎬ unless a transport
swab ⎭ medium is used.

3. Due to the protective vaginal acidity vaginal discharge and inflammation are not caused, in the first instance, by the ordinary pyogenic organisms (e.g. staphylococci, streptococci, *E. coli,* etc.): they may, however, be secondary invaders. The gonococcus is an exception.

Table 1. Causes of Vaginal Discharge

	Monilia Albicans (vaginal thrush)	Trichomonas vaginalis	Gonorrhoea	Cervical leucorrhoea
Nature	A yeast	A flagellate protozoon a little larger than a leucocyte	A Gram-negative diplococcus	Not an infective condition. It is merely an excess of mucus from the mucus-producing glands of the cervix
Symptoms	Irritation with or without discharge The consort may also suffer from penile irritation	Discharge with or without soreness The consort may harbour the organism without, however, suffering any ill-effects	Discharge and soreness often severe	Discharge with or without soreness
Appearance	White patches on the vaginal wall—'cream cheese' or 'cotton wool' appearance. The vaginal epithelium usually looks healthy between the patches	A greenish-yellow, frothy, watery discharge. The vaginal epithelium may look red and sore	A thick yellow purulent discharge. The vaginal epithelium is very inflamed	A clear or white, thick, mucoid discharge. The vaginal wall has its normal healthy pink colour
Investigation	A vaginal swab is sent to the laboratory where a smear is made and stained by Gram's method. The report can be given at once. (Confirmation by culture, however, takes longer.)	A vaginal swab is sent at once to the laboratory where the material is diluted with saline (1 drop), the motile organisms being directly visible without staining. The report can be given at	A urethral and an endocervical swab are sent to the laboratory for culture. Microscopy is performed on the culture. The report will not be available for at least 48 hours	

A cervical smear is an excellent method of detecting both *Trichomonas* and *Monilia*

	If the swab cannot reach the laboratory within half an hour there is no satisfactory method of detecting the organism with any degree of certainty	If the laboratory is not nearby, the swabs are placed in a tube containing a transport medium. This is a fluid which preserves the gonococcus in culture until the laboratory is reached	Local toilet; bathe with plain water (no antiseptics and little soap) and use powder lavishly. Wear (*a*) loose-fitting absorbant panties (i.e. cotton not nylon), and (*b*) clothes allowing good ventilation, e.g. open tights and skirts rather than trousers. No other treatment is possible or necessary
Treatment	1. Clotrimazole (Canestan) vaginal tablets (100 mg) each night for 6 nights 2. Nystatin pessaries each night for 2 weeks (100,000 units each) 3. Clotrimazole cream or Nystatin cream to consort in cases of recurrence or failure to respond. Apply to penis, scrotal and perianal area.	1. Metronidazole (Flagyl), 200 mg tds by mouth for 1 week. If necessary the consort may also receive the same course (contra-indicated in the first 3 months of pregnancy). 2. Acetarsol Pessary (SVC pessary), one or two per night for at least one month. This treatment has been largely supplanted by metronidazole.	Penicillin injections under the supervision of a venereologist e.g. aqueous procaine penicillin 2·4 megaunits im: preceded by probenecid 1 g by mouth.	

5 Retrodisplacement of the Uterus

Retroflexion	A backward angulation of the corpus on the cervix.
Retroversion	The whole uterus is tilted backwards, i.e. the cervix points forward of the vaginal axis.
Infertility and Recurrent Abortion	Rarely caused by retrodisplacement of the uterus, according to the most recent evidence.
Incarceration of the Retroflexed or Retroverted Gravid Uterus	**Sequence of Events** **1.** The fundus of the growing uterus fails to escape past the sacral promontory, due to adhesions, or an overhanging promontory. **2.** The uterus, growing in the pelvis, presses on the bladder causing *partial retention* and *frequency.* **3.** The cervix is forced forwards against the symphysis pubis, pressing on the urethra, elongating it and causing obstruction. This leads to *acute retention* and then to *retention with overflow.* **4.** The distended bladder presses the fundus still deeper into the pelvis, setting up a vicious circle.

80

5. If ignored or neglected the possible sequelae are:

a. Severe urinary infection with gangrene or rupture of the bladder.

b. Uraemia due to renal back-pressure.

c. Sacculation of the uterus—very rare.

Incidence of the Condition. Very rare. Retrodisplacement of the uterus, however, is found in 20% of the population; it follows, therefore, that the fundus usually escapes above the promontory during pregnancy, so there is little justification for correcting retrodisplacements of the uterus discovered accidentally in early pregnancy.

Time of Onset of Urinary Symptoms. Twelfth week of pregnancy.

Treatment. Admit to hospital, insert an indwelling catheter, emptying the bladder and allowing it to continue to drain into a bottle. The uterus will rise from the pelvis spontaneously once the vicious circle is broken. *N.B.*

a. Slow decompression is now no longer considered necessary in most centres: the dangers of urinary suppression and haematuria being more theoretical than real.

b. Active measures to replace the uterus are seldom required.

Retro-displace-ment at the Postnatal Clinic

1. Most of the symptoms attributed to retrodisplacement in the past, e.g. menorrhagia, mid-sacral backache, dysmenorrhoea, etc., are no longer held by the majority of gynaecologists to be so caused. Only *deep dyspareunia* can confidently be blamed on a retrodisplacement of the uterus.

2. Correction of a retrodisplacement and holding the uterus forward by a Hodge pessary is only likely to have a temporary effect, i.e. so long as the pessary is in situ.

Therefore:

1. Regard a retroverted or retroflexed position of the uterus as being a physiological one until proved otherwise.

2. Most people have given up the correction of retrodisplacement at the postnatal clinic.

3. Never tell a woman that she has a 'misplaced womb'. She may develop symptoms as soon as she is aware of the displacement.

Hyperemesis Gravidarum

AETIOLOGY

1. The basic cause is unknown, as is the cause of 'physiological' vomiting of pregnancy.
2. Psychological factors, however, play a part in aggravating the condition. An over-attentive mother or mother-in-law is a common finding.
3. It is common in the presence of *hydatidiform mole*.

N.B. There is no evidence for a specific 'toxin' as the cause, although the patient may become toxic as the result of severe vomiting. Therefore, it is a bad policy to include hyperemesis under the general heading of 'toxaemias of pregnancy'; it may suggest associations, e.g. with pre-eclampsia, which are not proved or intended.

CLINICALLY

1. Begins as 'physiological' morning sickness and then becomes worse until there is vomiting after every meal. The patient can become dangerously ill and dehydrated.
2. Usually passes off spontaneously by 16 weeks' gestation.
3. Vomiting may occur for the first time, or

recur late in pregnancy. There may be an underlying cause sometimes, e.g. hiatus hernia, but most cases respond to treatment as for the vomiting of early pregnancy.

DIAGNOSIS

Other causes of vomiting must not be forgotten:
1. Peptic ulceration.
2. Appendicitis.
3. Severe pre-eclampsia (in later pregnancy).
4. Infective hepatitis.
5. Hiatus hernia (in later pregnancy).
6. Intestinal obstruction.
7. Acute pyelitis.

TREATMENT

Mild Cases

Dietetic Advice
1. 'Little and often'. Six small meals a day.
2. Eat meals dry and drink between.
3. Choose whatever food is fancied.

Drugs
The doctor may order one of a variety of drugs, e.g.:
1. Promethazine hydrochloride (Phenergan) 50 mg nocte; or
2. Ancoloxin tabs i mane, tabs ii nocte.

Severe Cases

Ketosis or clinical dehydration is present.

General
1. Admit to hospital.
2. Isolate if possible.
3. No visitors until vomiting has ceased for 24 hours.
4. No vomit bowl on display near the bed.
5. A kind but not over-sympathetic attitude.
6. Try to solve home or domestic problems.

Diet

1. Nothing by mouth until vomiting has ceased for 24 hours. During this time intravenous glucose or saline-glucose will be ordered. (Glucose-saline should be maintained until chlorides reappear in the urine—in severe vomiting they will have been absent.)
2. Gradually wean back to oral feeding by small quantities of fluids, reverting, however, to the stricter régime if vomiting recommences.
3. *Thiamine hydrochloride* (Vitamin B₁) 100 mg by injection in severe cases to avoid Wernicke's encephalopathy.

Observations

1. Accurate fluid balance sheet.
N.B. Express all quantities in ml.
Make the beginning and end of the 24-hr period clear and add up the totals for that period.
2. Maternal pulse and temperature.
3. Blood pressure twice daily.
4. All specimens of urine to be tested for: Albumin; Ketones; Chlorides.

7   Pre-eclampsia

DEFINITION

Pre-eclampsia is a condition peculiar to pregnancy which in its fully developed form is characterized by *hypertension, oedema* and *albuminuria.*
N.B. With adequate antenatal care the disease should be detected almost always before albuminuria appears.

CAUSE

Processes Present in Pre-eclampsia and Eclampsia

Angiospasm. Causing:
a. Hypertension
b. In the kidney (i) reversible renal damage leading to *proteinuria;* (ii) *Bilateral renal cortical necrosis* or *lower nephron nephrosis* with anuria (*see* p. 111).
c. Epileptiform fits in eclampsia.
The hypertensive agent is *not known.*

Oedema. Due to:
a. Retention of sodium and water in the body.
b. Some electrolyte shift osmotically attracting fluid into the intra-cellular space
Either or both (evidence is conflicting).

This is aggravated by a low serum protein when proteinuria is present.

Disseminated Intravascular Coagulation is reported as occurring in pre-eclampsia and eclampsia and it may be the cause of the *liver* and *renal changes* as well as producing serious *pulmonary complications* with respiratory failure. A falling platelet count warns that disseminated intravascular coagulation is occurring.

The Basic Trigger Mechanism

This is not known but the following factors have to be taken into account by any theory:
1. Pre-eclampsia occurs mainly in *first pregnancies*. When it occurs in a later pregnancy it is usually with a *new consort:* this gives support to a view that the condition may be an autoimmune response to fetal antigens.
2. It is more common with *twins*.
3. There is a high incidence with *hydatidiform mole*.
4. Eclamptic fits may occur for the first time after delivery.

DANGERS

Maternal

Immediate (*see Table,* p. 90)
1. Cerebral haemorrhage (the commonest cause of death in pre-eclampsia).
2. Accidental haemorrhage, leading to fatal shock, postpartum haemorrhage and/or anuria.
3. Eclampsia with a 5% mortality, q.v.
4. Anuria—either with severe pre-eclampsia or after eclampsia or accidental haemorrhage.
5. Liver failure with jaundice in severe pre-eclampsia as in eclampsia, q.v.
6. Hypertensive heart failure ⎫
7. Retinal haemorrhage.   ⎬ rare.
                                ⎭

Remote. Permanently raised blood pressure. Some authorities doubt whether pre-eclampsia can lead to this. Perhaps it merely causes permanent hypertension to appear, in those who are predisposed to that condition by heredity, earlier than it would otherwise have done.

Fetal

1. Accidental haemorrhage (leading to placental separation).
2. Placental insufficiency due to spasm of placental vessels. (Infarcts are often seen.)
3. Prematurity:
a. Premature delivery is often effected in the fetal as well as the maternal interest, but the risks of prematurity and of the induction have to be weighed against the risk of continued intra-uterine life.
b. Placental insufficiency leads to smaller babies in pre-eclamptic pregnancies.
4. Intra-uterine infection (occasionally follows surgical induction of labour).

IMPORTANCE

Although for many years the maternal deaths from the pre-eclampsia, eclampsia and essential hypertension group of conditions outnumbered any other group of causes of maternal death, e.g. 'sepsis', 'haemorrhage' or 'abortion', since 1958 improved standards of antenatal care had resulted in such a fall in maternal deaths from the hypertensive diseases of pregnancy that they had fallen to third place in order of importance by 1972. By 1975, however, they had again risen to first place, due largely to the fall in deaths from abortion; in the latest available figures deaths from hypertensive diseases of pregnancy rank second only to deaths from pulmonary embolism. It is true that the number of women dying from pre-eclampsia and eclampsia has fallen steadily over the years, but so has the number from the other causes of maternal death. Nevertheless, many women die annually from these conditions: the relative importance of the various causes of maternal death can best be studied by reference to the *Report on Confidential Enquiries into Maternal Death.* * A table is shown compiled from the 1976–78 Report (*see* p. 90).

EARLY DETECTION OF PRE-ECLAMPSIA

Object

1. If pre-eclampsia is detected early (i.e. before albuminuria appears), it is usually reversible by rest, sedatives and salt-free diet, so that pregnancy can be carried on with safety to mother and baby.

2. Once it has become severe (albumin present), or rapidly advancing, it is usually only a matter of days at the most before the pregnancy must be terminated in the interest of both mother and baby, with, however, the hazard of prematurity.

First Signs of Pre-eclampsia

Rise of Blood Pressure

1. *Some Observations on Blood Pressure.*

a. Blood pressure is not something which can be measured like a piece of string and given a definite and inflexible length. It tends to vary from moment to moment to a greater or lesser degree, rising with excitement or activity and settling on rest. In this it resembles a piece of elastic which can be measured at full stretch or at rest.

The significance of any one reading, therefore, depends not only on the recorded level but on the condition of the patient at the time of recording. A pressure which rises considerably with stimulus is said to be *labile.*

*Department of Health and Social Security (1982) *Reports on Health and Social Subjects, No. 26, Report on Confidential Enquiries into Maternal Deaths in England and Wales,* 1976–78, London, HMSO.

Causes of Maternal Death in England and Wales
1976–1978

Pulmonary Embolism			45
Hypertensive diseases of pregnancy			
Eclampsia	8		
Cerebral haemorrhage			
Cerebral oedema	2		
Asphyxia	1		
Anoxic cardiac arrest	1		
Unknown	1	13	
Pre-eclampsia			
Cerebral haemorrhage	9		
Anoxic cardiac arrest	2		
Hepatorenal failure	1		
Others	4	16	29
Haemorrhage			
Accidental	6	(5 with coagulation disorder)	
Placenta praevia	2		
Post-partum haemorrhage	18	(1 with inversion of the uterus)	26
Abortion			
Illegal	4		
Spontaneous	3	(including 1 due to anaesthesia)	
Legal	12	(including 4 due to anaesthesia)	
			19
Other Causes			
Anaesthesia	24		
(excluding operations for abortion and ectopic pregnancy)			
Ectopic pregnancy	22	(including 1 due to anaesthesia)	
Sepsis (excluding abortion)	17		
Ruptured uterus	14		
Amniotic fluid embolism (histologically proven)	11		
Miscellaneous	20		108
			227

b. Ideally, a full blood pressure recording should give:

The *basal level,* i.e. the lowest reading obtained under conditions of complete rest or even under sedation.

The *highest level* to which it can be raised by stimulus. In practice it would be too complicated to do this as a routine procedure.

c. Some idea of the lability of a person's blood pressure can be obtained by:

Studying a series of recordings over several visits, or:

Repeating the recording at any one visit, e.g.: (i) At the first visit to the clinic, excitement makes the labile blood pressure rise (Browne's 'early warning rise'); (ii) Sometimes the patient will arrive after hurrying and a higher record will be achieved; (iii) If a pressure to be taken again by the midwife, a previously high reading may return, after rest, to a lower level. But if attention be drawn to the finding, particularly if a doctor be asked to repeat it, a higher reading than the original one may be obtained, the labile quality being thus revealed.

N.B. It cannot be too strongly emphasized that the highest reading obtained must be recorded as this is the important danger signal. The common practice of repeating the reading, and then, if it be a lower one, recording this only, is to 'play the ostrich' and to mislead the obstetrician. *Always record the highest as well as the lowest reading.*

d. The blood pressure tends to fall during the middle trimester, so if a reading is not obtained in the first trimester, an intrinsically labile pressure may be missed until it is made manifest later in pregnancy when it cannot easily be distinguished from pre-eclampsia.

e. Patients with a labile pressure (or with fixed hypertension) are much more likely to get pre-eclampsia later in pregnancy than those where pressure is stable and consistently below the upper limit of normal.

2. *Significance of a Rise of Blood Pressure*
a. The 'normal' pressure for obstetrical purposes is one which does not exceed 130/80. (Browne took a stricter level still, viz. 120/80.) However, the basal level must be taken into account: a rise of 20 mmHg over the basal systolic pressure must be regarded as significant, for obstetric purposes: (1) 135/85, whatever the basal pressure, or (2) 130/80, when the basal pressure was 110/70, are both examples of abnormal blood pressure.
b. A 'new' rise of pressure after the 24th week may be either impending pre-eclampsia or the manifestation of a labile blood pressure hitherto concealed. In practice it is better to regard it as the former and to take steps accordingly (*see below*), or an opportunity to prevent a severe pre-eclampsia may be missed. Nevertheless, when the rise affects the systolic pressure alone, in the absence of oedema and albuminuria, it is more likely to be the result of a labile hypertension.
c. Where pre-eclampsia has developed, a rise of blood pressure (by the standards given above) will almost invariably have occurred before oedema or albuminuria.

Water Retention
1. *Oedema* may occasionally be the first sign of impending pre-eclampsia.
a. Water retention to some extent is physiological in pregnancy and there is no sharp dividing line between this and the pathological retention of pre-eclampsia; one merges imperceptibility into the other.
b. Swelling of the feet and ankles is assisted by gravity and indeed can sometimes occur in the non-pregnant person after long standing.
c. Oedema of the fingers, however, manifested by an increased tightness of the wedding ring, must be regarded as pathological and an important warning sign even without a rise of blood pressure. It is also a reliable finding if the patient is questioned intelligently; probably

more reliable than weight gain, which is open to error (q.v.), and certainly less time-consuming.
2. *Abnormal Weight Gain, Showing Occult Oedema*
a. Normal gain averages 1·8 kg per month in the last half of pregnancy; thus a monthly gain of over 2 kg may be regarded as abnormal.
b. Value in Prediction:
Fifty per cent of cases gaining more than 2·27 kg (5 lb) in a month developed pre-eclampsia.
0·9% of cases with *no* excessive weight gain developed pre-eclampsia.

Sixty-five per cent of cases of pre-eclampsia showed an abnormal weight gain as the first sign (Arwyn Evans*).

Thus only half of the cases of abnormal weight gain actually develop pre-eclampsia, but very few cases whose gain is within normal limits do so.
c. Results. Hamlin of Sydney recorded the weight gain in all patients between the 20th and 30th weeks, those exceeding 3·63 kg (8 lb) gain in this period were followed up carefully and put on a salt-free and low carbohydrate diet. He had no case of eclampsia in the next 8000 deliveries following the institution of the régime. (Previously the rate had been 1 case of eclampsia to every 350 booked cases delivered.)
d. Sources of Error: (1) Physiological diurnal variations (bowels, bladder, food, etc.) (2) Variations due to clothing. (3) Variations due to scales. (4) Weight change due to other factors, such as fat deposition or removal. (The frequent advocacy of carbohydrate-restricted diet increases this error.)

Albuminuria
1. This is hardly ever the first sign of pre-eclampsia. If the blood pressure appears to be normal, a repeated test will usually show a

*Evans M. D. Arwyn (1937) *Br. Med. J.* **1**, 157.

raised reading if in the end it proves to be due to pre-eclampsia.

2. *Investigation and Differential Diagnosis if Blood Pressure is Normal*

a. Present in ordinary specimen, but *absent in mid-stream specimen—vaginal discharge.*

b. Present in mid-stream specimen, too: (1) Urinary tract infection—acute cystitis or pyelitis. (2) Glomerulonephritis. (3) Chronic pyelonephritis, with or without stones. (4) Renal tuberculosis. (5) Orthostatic albuminuria. (6) Unexplained cases. (7) Accompanying obvious severe disease, e.g. anaemia, cardiac conditions, etc.

N.B. Common causes of albuminuria in pregnancy are: (1) Pre-eclampsia and essential hypertension. (2) Vaginal discharge. (3) Urinary tract infections.

TYPES OF CASE TO WATCH CLOSELY

1. Primigravidae. Seventy per cent of pre-eclamptics are primigravidae.

2. 'Grand multips'.

3. Twin pregnancies.

4. Cases with (a) Labile blood pressures (including the 'early warning rise' cases) (b) Fixed hypertension.

5. Those with a history of a previous early and severe pre-eclampsia, e.g. at 28 weeks, or of previous accidental haemorrhage.

6. Diabetics.

MANAGEMENT

Of cases whose blood pressure had been 'normal' in early pregnancy.

At Clinic **Admit to Hospital** cases with:
1. Blood pressure equal to or exceeding 140 mm systolic.

2. Blood pressure exceeding 130/80 mm with oedema of the fingers or abnormal weight gain.
3. Albuminuria, unless: (1) mid-stream specimen of urine clear; (2) blood pressure normal; and (3) no oedema of fingers.

Observe at the Clinic weekly (or even more often), cases showing:
1. Blood pressure (1) Exceeding 130/80; or (2) Exceeding basal systolic level by 20 mmHg or more.
2. Oedema; especially of fingers.
3. Weight gain of more than 2 kg in a month (or any shorter period).
N.B. See a case as often as is required, irrespective of the routine for that period of gestation. Sometimes a home visit by the district midwife, armed with a sphygmomanometer, will help.

Régime
1. Rest at home.
2. Sedation, if required.
3. Cardiff 'kick charts' may be useful as a warning to seek advice.

On Ward

Observations
1. Blood *pressure recording.*
a. Four-hourly in mildest cases, reverting to twice daily in a few days.
b. Quarter-hourly in very severe cases, as for an eclamptic.
c. Intermediate frequency of recording may be ordered.
2. Daily Esbach estimation of *proteinuria.*
3. Record progress of *oedema* daily.
4. Examine a *mid-stream specimen of urine* for pus cells. (The albumin may be due to urinary infection even if the blood pressure be raised.)
5. *Fluid balance* chart for moderate and severe cases.
6. *The retina* is examined once a week.
7. Tests for *fetal growth* and *placental*

function. (*see* under 'Growth Retardation', p. 56).

a. Urinary or blood *oestriol estimation.*

b. *Ultrasonography,* i.e. (1) biparietal diameter; and/or (2) abdominal circumference.

N.B. Both (*a*) and (*b*) are recorded on a graph for it is the serial observations which are important: no action would be taken on a single low reading.

c. *Fetal cardiotocography.*

8. The *lecithin/sphingomyelin ratio* may indicate when delivery would be reasonably safe for the baby in cases where some degree of prematurity is involved.

Régime

1. Complete bed rest to begin with; gradual ambulation as condition improves in mild cases.

2. Sedation may be needed on admission for severe cases but is best avoided in milder cases, at least for 24 hours to see if the blood pressure falls on rest alone.

a. Amylobarbitone 200 mg, 8-hourly to 3-hourly, or

b. Diazepam 2–5 mg, tds.

3. Hypotensive drugs. In general these are disappointing for the management of pre-eclampsia but may be tried in moderately severe cases.

a. Methyldopa 250 mg, bd or tds; adjust upwards at intervals of 2 days.

b. Severe cases treat as for eclampsia.

Outcome

1. *Mild Cases*

The condition is restored to normal and the patient goes home to rest and continue with weekly observation at antenatal clinic.

2. *Severe Cases*

Those which do not revert to normal eventually need terminating by artificial rupture of the membranes (or even by Caesarean section, especially if under 36 weeks). Forceps extraction at full dilatation is desirable unless a quick spontaneous delivery is anticipated.

PRE-ECLAMPTIC STATE

Definition

A severe case of pre-eclampsia having, in addition, the symptoms of headaches, spots in front of the eyes, facial twitching, epigastric pain and vomiting.

Management

Treat as an eclamptic, for she is liable to have a fit at any minute. The case must be sedated at once and *never left, until handed over to hospital staff.* The 'Flying Squad' should be called out.

N.B. Treat such a case as a grave emergency.

Eclampsia

DEFINITION

A case of pre-eclampsia with superimposed *epileptiform fits.*
N.B. If there has been no fit it is not eclampsia, regardless of the pathological findings.

PATHOLOGY

Liver

Areas of haemorrhage interspersed with necrotic patches. These findings may occur in severe cases of pre-eclampsia.

Kidney

1. *Cases without Anuria:* Certain changes are seen in the glomerular capillaries (thickening of the basement membrane and swelling of the endothelial cells).
2. *Cases with Anuria:*
a. Bilateral renal cortical necrosis.
b. Lower nephron nephrosis.

DIFFERENTIAL DIAGNOSIS OF FITS

1. Hysteria.
2. Epilepsy: (*a*) The signs of pre-eclampsia are absent; (*b*) History of previous fits.
3. Strychnine poisoning.
4. Syncope.

PROGNOSIS

Maternal

Five per cent mortality. Some centres have better figures, some worse.
Causes of death. See Table in previous chapter, p. 90.
Eclampsia is followed by a very high incidence of *permanently raised blood pressure.*
Temporary paresis, due to cerebral angiospasm, may accompany or follow the disease.

Fetal

Five per cent mortality.
Causes of death.
1. Prematurity.
2. Asphyxia:
a. Accidental haemorrhage.
b. Placental insufficiency.
c. Maternal anoxia.
d. Drugs given to mother interfering with respiration after birth.
3. Pneumonia due to intra-uterine sepsis.
4. Injuries at delivery.

Signs of Poor Prognosis

1. Fits exceed ten in number.
2. Patient remains in coma between fits.
3. Blood pressure remains high between fits, and exceeds 200.
4. Maternal pulse rises and exceeds 120.
5. Pyrexia.
6. Moist lungs and cyanosis.
7. Development of anuria or oliguria,

particularly if preceded by a small quantity of bloodstained urine.

8. A falling platelet count indicating disseminated intravascular coagulation.

TREATMENT

Prophylactic
See under
'Pre-
eclampsia',
Chapter 7

The most common type of eclampsia seen nowadays is the single fit occurring at full dilatation or after delivery: these cases are not always in known pre-eclamptics. These can only be prevented by more frequent blood pressure observations in labour and in the first 6 days of the puerperium, paying especial attention to the 'rebound' which is common on about the 4th day. (Many people say that fits occurring after 48 hours from delivery are not true eclampsia.)

Therapeutic

General Measures
a. Continuous supervision, especially: (i) to prevent injury during a fit, and (ii) to maintain the airway.
b. Avoid external stimuli, e.g. (i) loud noise, (ii) bright lights—nevertheless adequate light to observe the patient especially for cyanosis, (iii) moving the patient, except when sedated.
c. Have available (i) a padded gag, (ii) a pharyngeal airway, (iii) oxygen mask.
d. Continuous bladder drainage.
e. Intravenous line.

Observations
a. Maternal (i) blood pressure, (ii) pulse, (iii) respirations—quarter-hourly.
b. Fetal heart rate—continuously or at least quarter-hourly.
c. Maternal temperature—frequently.
d. Fluid balance, i.e. (i) fluid intake, (ii) urinary output hourly.
e. Depth of sedation.
f. Presence, strength and frequency of contractions.

First Aid Measures

a. Call the Obstetric Flying Squad if outside a major obstetric unit. They should accompany the patient to hospital if she is not already there.

b. Diazepam (Valium) 5–10 mg by slow i.v. bolus injection.

c. Hydralazine (Apresoline) 10–20 mg by slow i.v. bolus injection.

If these drugs are not available the following can be used: (i) Morphia 15–30 mg i.v. or, (ii) Paraldehyde 5–10 ml i.m. (not in a plastic syringe).

Maintenance Measures

1. *Anticonvulsant Therapy*

a. *Chlormethiazole* (Heminevrin) by continuous i.v. infusion; 0·8% solution at 60 drops/min, *initially* to make the patient drowsy but rousable. *Continue* with 10–15 drops/min; normal daily dose is 6–8 g.

Drip rate of 10 d.p.m. gives 1 g in 3 hours;
Drip rate of 15 d.p.m. gives 1 g in 2 hours;
Drip rate of 30 d.p.m. gives 1 g in 1 hour.
or

b. *Diazepam* 30 mg in 5% dextrose

Give 5–10 mg/hour and not more than 40 mg in 4 hours or 60 mg in 24 hours.

N.B. It is accumulative and depresses fetal respirations.

c. *Full relaxant anaesthesia* if fits are uncontrolled.

2. *Hypotensive Therapy*

Many different preparations are in use for this purpose and there is no agreement as to the best one to employ.

Some suggestions are:

a. *Hydralazine* (Apresoline) 10–20 mg i.v. by slow bolus injection: repeat as necessary, maximum 200 mg/day.

N.B. (1) It is unstable in solution; do not give by continuous infusion. (2) Do not give in a dextrose solution.

b. *Labetalol (Trandate)* 200 mg diluted with 200 ml dextrose-saline. 2 ml/min until response is obtained. Maximum dose 200 mg.

Analgesia
a. Epidural blockade is preferable where possible, otherwise:
b. Pethidine 25 mg i.v., repeated as required but remember there is a cumulative respiratory depressant effect.

Additional Measures

1. *Mannitol*
Use. To attract fluid from the extracellular compartment into the intravascular compartment osmotically to: (i) reduce cerebral oedema and help to reduce the incidence of fits, (ii) promote diuresis.
Indications. (i) Urinary output less than 40 ml/hour. (ii) Central venous pressure less than 5 cm H_2O.
Danger. If given without a low CVP (i.e. when there may be renal failure), water intoxication may result (*see below* under Anuria).
Dosage. 1 g/kg in a 25% solution over 30 min (precede by a test dose of 200 mg/kg).

2. *Magnesium Sulphate*
10 ml of 25% i.v. (over 5 min). Lowers blood pressure. The face feels and is flushed during injection.

3. *Spinal Anaesthesia*
Spinal anaesthesia lowers blood pressure by sympathetic block. May be useful when other measures fail.

Delivery. In general, vaginal delivery should be aimed at as being better tolerated than a major operation, such as Caesarean section, in a patient whose cardiac condition is already compromised by the eclamptic situation; but if delivery is likely to be long delayed, abdominal delivery should be performed. In any case, forceps extraction should be performed, preferably under general anaesthesia, when reasonably possible.
Warning Signs Demanding Early Delivery are:
a. Rising maternal pulse rate.

b. Pulmonary congestion and respiratory difficulty.
c. A falling platelet count.
d. Uncontrollable blood pressure.
e. Hepatic failure.
f. Renal failure.

Management of Anuria. As soon as it is apparent that the urinary output is reduced the following régime must be instituted:

1. Keep a very careful *fluid-balance chart.*

2. *Restrict total fluid intake* to 500 ml plus the previous day's urinary output. This is based on the assumption that 1000 ml is all the fluid the body can dispose of by what is called the 'insensible loss', viz., from lungs and skin, and that 500 ml of water is produced by metabolism. If more fluid than this is given the patient becomes 'waterlogged' and her chances of survival are reduced.

3. Give up to 200 g of glucose daily in the above fluid. No protein is given as this will cause the blood urea to rise while the kidneys are out of action.

This solution, which may be 40% glucose, is very syrupy and sweet and can be given:

a. As a fruit drink, or

b. By gastric 'drip', or

c. As a 'drip' into the inferior vena cava, using a polythene catheter threaded upwards through the internal saphenous vein (in Scarpa's triangle) into the femoral and external iliac veins. A 20% solution is preferable.

4. *Daily blood electrolyte estimations* are necessary and variations from normal may need correction by adjusting the transfused fluids or the use of ion-exchange resins.

5. A falling haemoglobin will need blood *transfusion.*

6. Renal dialysis should be used, with any of the following indications:

a. Clinical deterioration.

b. A blood urea of over 65 mmol/l.

c. Severe acidosis.

d. A rising blood potassium.

7. Careful *barrier nursing and aseptic precautions.* These cases are very liable to infection. A single injection of ampicillin may be given as a prophylactic: such a dose will probably act for a week as it is not being excreted.

By these techniques the patient can be kept alive until the kidneys start functioning again, if the damage has not been too great for this to occur.

N.B. Anuria is a complication of:

1. Eclampsia, severe pre-eclampsia.

2. Severe concealed accidental haemorrhage.

3. Mismatched blood transfusion.

4. Severe trauma, e.g.

a. Crushing of a limb ('Crush syndrome').

b. Serious operative procedures.

9 Essential Hypertension

NATURE

1. A raised blood pressure with no obvious organic cause.
2. It is inherited as a Mendelian dominant.

DIAGNOSIS

A raised blood pressure in the first trimester. A normal record in the second trimester is of little use as the pressure falls in the middle three months.

TYPES

Labile Blood Pressure

1. Rises on effort, excitement, etc., and falls to within normal limits at rest.
2. A precursor of the fixed hypertension.

Fixed Hypertension

This has a permanently raised basal level, but it may rise on stimulus to greater heights. Alternatively, it may be stable, varying little with stimulus.

DANGERS

Superadded

a. Pre-eclampsia. Seven times more common than in the normotensive woman.
b. Eclampsia. Ten times more common than in the normotensive woman.

Others

All the other dangers listed in Chapter 7 apply here, too, but are much more common if pre-eclampsia is superadded.
Note: When proteinuria appears in pure essential hypertension (which it tends to do when the systolic pressure reaches approximately 160 mmHg), then (i) accidental haemorrhage, or (ii) fetal death from placental insufficiency is imminent.

MANAGEMENT

Objects of Antenatal Care

1. To prevent delay or detect the onset of pre-eclampsia.
2. To oppose the tendency of the blood pressure to rise towards term with the danger of:
a. Accidental haemorrhage.
b. Fetal death from placental insufficiency.

Admission for Assessment

1. Admit for assessment when first seen at antenatal clinic unless a very mild case.
2. Observe blood pressure 4-hourly and for at least 24 hours without treatment.
3. Sedation—at night if not sleeping and in daytime if anxious or highly strung, e.g. (i) diazepam 2–5 mg tds, or (ii) sodium amytal 200 mg up to 4-hourly (depending on severity of case).
4. Methyldopa (other hypotensive drugs also in use), 250 mg tds. Increase as required by 250 mg steps at intervals of not less than 2

days. Maximum dose 1 g tds though this dose is seldom required.

5. If control is established the patient is discharged to observation at clinic frequently, and in any case weekly from 28th week.

Serial Observations on the Fetal Wellbeing
see under 'Growth Retardation'

1. *Biparietal diameter* (or other ultrasound observation, e.g. abdominal circumference) every 2 weeks from 28th week.
2. *Oestriol levels,* e.g. urinary oestriol/creatinine ratio every 2 weeks from 34th week.
3. *Kick chart.*
4. *Cardiotocography* (this can be done at the clinic).

Further Observations on Mother

1. Blood pressure (modify the dose of hypotensive drug if required).
2. Test urine for protein.
3. Presence of finger oedema or excessive weight gain.

Readmission

Indications
1. Deterioration of any of the fetal well-being parameters.
2. Failure to control the blood pressure.
3. Appearance of proteinuria.
4. Development of finger oedema or excessive weight gain.

Observations—continued on ward.

Outcome
1. If condition stabilizes—discharge from hospital may be offered.
2. If not—keep till delivered.

Delivery

Timing
When it is considered that the risks of premature delivery are outweighed by those of continued intra-uterine existence, i.e. of the risk of fetal death in utero.

The lecithin/sphingomyelin index may assist in making the decision.

Method
1. Induction of labour as a rule.
2. Elective Caesarean section if (i) the fetal danger is great, (ii) it is very premature when it is difficult to get the patient into labour.

Antepartum Haemorrhage

CLASSIFICATION

Accidental Haemorrhage (*abruptio placentae*)

Bleeding after the 28th week of pregnancy from the placental site situated wholly on the upper segment.

Inevitable Haemorrhage

(Bleeding from a separated placenta praevia) Bleeding after the 28th week of pregnancy from the placental site situated wholly or partially on the lower segment.

Vaginal and Cervical Causes of Bleeding

1. Vascular erosion.
2. Cervical polyp.
3. Varicosities of the cervix.
4. Carcinoma of the cervix.
5. Urethral caruncle.

ACCIDENTAL HAEMORRHAGE (Abruptio Placentae)

Aetiology

1. Pre-eclampsia, essential hypertension, or chronic nephritis. It is evident that these factors do not play as important a role in the aetiology of accidental haemorrhage as was thought at

one time: they play a part probably in about only 25% of cases.

2. Trauma—usually external version, especially under anaesthesia. Blows on the abdomen are unlikely to lead to haemorrhage unless severe.

3. Short cord—rare.

4. Folic-acid deficiency. Recent work suggests this as a factor.

5. Unknown causes. Some of these, especially the mild cases, may be due to bleeding from:

a. The lower edge of a placenta lying low in the upper segment, though not reaching the lower segment when it would be placenta praevia.

b. The endometrium or decidua.

Pathology

Revealed. All the blood escapes per vaginam. One presumes that in these cases if the bleeding is from the placental site it will be from the inferior margin of a low lying placenta (though not on the lower segment). Alternatively, it may be from the decidua.

Concealed

1. The blood collects as *retroplacental blood clot.*

2. In severe cases not only has the placenta been stripped completely off the uterine wall by the clot but the whole uterine wall is infiltrated with blood giving a subperitoneal 'bruise' or discoloration. This type of uterus is called the '*Couvelaire uterus*'. (The cause for this is uncertain but it may be due to clotting defect.)

3. *Clotting defect* may lead to continued bleeding and subsequent postpartum haemorrhage:

Causes

FIBRINOGEN DEPLETION.

The *massive clotting process* has used up large amounts of fibrinogen which is not being replaced by the liver, the function of which is depressed by the poor circulation resulting from the shock which is present.

Thromboplastins from the damaged uterine wall and placenta are absorbed and lead to increased intravascular fibrin deposition which in turn is removed by a speeding up of the fibrinolytic process.

FIBRINOGEN DEGRADATION PRODUCTS. These degradation products interfere with the polymerization of fibrin monomer to fibrin polymer and result from the speeding up of the process of fibrinolysis acting on the intravascular fibrinogen-fibrin conversion. Plasmin, which produces fibrinolysis, is produced from plasminogen by the action of plasminogen activators which are absorbed from the damaged uterine tissue (*see* chart, p. 247).

4. *Anuria* may result due to:

a. Bilateral renal cortical necrosis, or

b. Lower nephron nephrosis.

It is brought about by the compensatory angiospasm and possibly, also, by other mechanisms which are not clearly understood.

Mixed. Very often both a concealed and a revealed element are present, but the management is determined by whichever factor predominates.

Clinical Presentation

Revealed

1. *Mild.* A simple small blood loss: it must be considered to be potentially a case of placenta praevia until investigation has excluded this. The fact that the fetal head is found well down into the pelvis may make placenta praevia less likely but does not completely exclude a minor degree.

2. *Severe.* Almost invariably diagnosed as placenta praevia bleeding. The absence of a low lying placenta will be discovered at the inevitable examination under anaesthesia or Caesarean section which will be required as a matter of urgency. The presenting part may be high or low (*see* last paragraph).

Concealed
1. *Mild.* A localized patch of tenderness over the uterus. The diagnosis is only presumptive.
2. *Severe*
a. Clinically shocked, though the blood pressure is often slightly raised due to the compensatory angiospasm.
b. The uterus is tender and 'wooden' due to uterine spasm. The fetal parts cannot be palpated.
c. The fetal heart is not heard.
d. There may be evidence of pre-existing pre-eclampsia, etc., but often there is not.
e. Anuria is common as a sequel.

Dangers

Maternal
1. Shock and death.
2. Postpartum haemorrhage due to clotting defect.
3. Anuria.

Fetal
1. Prematurity.
2. Death by immediate separation of the placenta.
3. Death by placental insufficiency after partial separation of the placenta.

Treatment

Mild (no shock)
1. If not near term:
a. Rest in bed for 4 days after the incident, unless the associated condition requires treatment for its own sake.
b. If there be a revealed element, investigate to exclude placenta praevia (*see below*).
c. Allow home ultimately.
d. Watch for fetal distress in labour and consider forceps extraction at full dilatation.
2. If 38 weeks or over, rupture the forewaters.

Severe

1. *Revealed*

Take to theatre as for a case of suspected praevia (*see below*).

a. Not in labour—Caesarean section.

b. In labour—rupture the forewaters; an oxytocic drip may be considered; blood transfusion.

2. *Concealed or mixed* (shock)

a. Treat shock by massive blood transfusion.

b. Rupture the forewaters.

c. Oxytocic drip.

d. If no result and condition deteriorates, Caesarean section, with or without hysterectomy, should be considered but the risks of clotting defect must be borne in mind.

e. Clotting defect (*see* under Postpartum haemorrhage, p. 237).

i. Detect

(i) Clinically by observing failure of blood to clot. (ii) By incubating plasma from 'at risk' case with thrombin to assess clot formation. If negative, repeat mixing the patient's plasma with some control plasma: if the result is still negative there is excess fibrinolysis present. (iii) By estimating the plasma fibrinogen. Less than 1 g/l/100 ml justifies therapy.

ii. Treat by:

(i) *Massive blood transfusion.* (ii) *Human fibrinogen* 5–8 g i.v. or quadruple strength plasma 500 ml (may supply other factors). (iii) *Antifibrinolytic agents:* Aprotinin (Trasylol) 500 000 KIU i.v. by slow injection within 30 min, then 50 000 KIU per hour by drip till haemostasis occurs, or Aminocaproic acid (Epsikapron) 5 g i.v., then 1 g per hour by i.v. drip till haemostasis occurs.

Theoretically, antifibrinolytic therapy might increase risk of pulmonary or renal thrombosis by opposing the mechanism for removing intravascular clot, in practice Aprotinin has been seen to work dramatically in arresting haemorrhage when all else has failed. (iv)

Heparin 1500 units per hour has been advocated to reduce the amount of intravascular clotting and hence the degree of fibrinolysis and the liberation of further fibrin degradation products which interfere with fibrin polymerization, but there might well be hesitation in using this form of therapy in a woman who is bleeding persistently.

iii. Other causes of clotting defect:
(i) Fetal death in utero for 3 weeks or more.
(ii) Amniotic embolism. (iii) Septic abortion.
f. Watch closely for *anuria* and treat it if it occurs (*see under* 'Eclampsia', pp. 103–104).

INEVITABLE HAEMORRHAGE (Placenta Praevia)

Cause of Bleeding	The inelastic placenta fails to keep pace with the stretching of the lower segment in late pregnancy or early labour.
Degrees	1st Degree Plasma dips on to the lower segment but not as low as the internal cervical os. (Lateral.) 2nd Degree The placental edge reaches to the margin of the internal os. (Marginal.) 3rd Degree The placenta covers the os before dilatation begins but would not do so at full dilatation. (Central.) 4th Degree The placenta would cover the os even at full dilatation. (Central.)

Comparison with Accidental Haemorrhage

	Inevitable	*Accidental*
Pain over uterus	Absent	Usually present
Palpation	Normal	Wooden, tender uterus with fetal parts not palpable in severe concealed variety; otherwise normal
Presenting part	High	May be engaged
Fetal heart	Usually heard	Absent in severe cases

Dangers

Maternal

1. *Haemorrhagic Shock.*

2. *The risks of Caesarean Section,* especially if the patient has already bled heavily. If there has been a previous Caesarean section the placenta may be very adherent to the scar; this may lead to uncontrollable bleeding requiring hysterectomy.

3. *Postpartum Haemorrhage*—the lower segment is not so efficient as the upper in controlling blood loss by the 'living ligature' action, therefore watch the delivered mother closely for some hours after delivery, especially after Caesarean section.

Fetal

1. *Placental Separation* leading to placental insufficiency.

2. *Pressure by the Baby on its own Placenta.*

3. *Fetal Death* following severe maternal collapse.

4. *Fetal Blood Loss from the Placenta,* spontaneously or on separating the placenta at Caesarean section, therefore observe the delivered baby closely for evidence of shock or anaemia.

5. *Prematurity,* when definitive treatment becomes obligatory due to haemorrhage or premature labour.

Procedure after admitting a Case of Antepartum Haemorrhage presumed to be due to Placenta Praevia

(Painless loss with a high presenting part.)

Under 38 Weeks

1. Put to bed:

a. Morphine.

b. Blood group and send serum to laboratory to be kept for an urgent demand.

c. Transfuse if necessary.

2. Inspect the cervix (after a few days) to exclude cervical causes of antepartum haemorrhage.

3. Examine the blood lost per vaginam for fetal blood.

4. Localize the placenta by ultrasonography.
5. If the placenta is found to be praevia, keep on the ward until 38 weeks.

With the tendency to diagnose placenta praevia by ultrasonography relatively early in pregnancy, e.g. under 28 weeks, there may be a case under certain circumstances for allowing the patient home after a good rest, readmitting at 34 weeks. The justification for this is:

a. A minor degree of placenta praevia early in pregnancy may cease to be a case of placenta praevia late in pregnancy.
b. A dangerous blood loss under 34 weeks from a minor degree of placenta praevia must be a very unlikely event.

It must be stated that this may be regarded as heresy by many, but sometimes heresy becomes accepted practice! If placenta praevia is excluded, the patient may be allowed home.
6. At 38 weeks take to theatre and examine under anaesthesia:
a. Everything must be ready for Caesarean section.
b. Blood, cross-matched, must be in theatre.
c. The anaesthetic should not start until everybody is 'scrubbed up'.
d. Degree 3 or 4—Caesarean section.

Degree 1 or 2, or no placenta felt—Rupture of Forewaters or Caesarean section according to: (i) the level and site of the placenta (posterior is less favourable than anterior); and (ii) whether the head will descend on to the placental edge.
N.B.   Even after ARM, watch for a few minutes to see if bleeding stops: Caesarean section may still be required. It is not always possible to explore the whole of the lower segment to exclude placenta praevia with certainty.
Exceptional cases
1. If the presenting part is so high, or the placentography report such that a central placenta praevia is almost certain, Caesarean

section should be performed without preliminary examination per vaginam.

2. The patient may have to go straight to theatre for EUA if:

a. Bleeding becomes dangerous—a heavy loss or a prolonged trickle.

b. If labour begins.

c. If there is marked fetal distress, particularly if the blood lost shows a significant amount of fetal blood. (If this should be observed, be on the watch for severe anaemia in the baby at delivery.)

38 Weeks or Over. Take the patient to theatre on admission and proceed as in 6, *above,* but bearing in mind the cases upon whom Caesarean section without preliminary vaginal examination is indicated.

Objects of the Conservative Treatment

The prognosis for the baby is improved by delaying definitive treatment, until the 38th week (it used to be the policy, until the early 40s, to take all cases of antepartum haemorrhage straight to theatre; the fetal loss from prematurity was high). It has proved possible to do this with safety to the mother provided that:

1. *No vaginal examination (other than with the speculum as mentioned) shall be done either before or after admission except as described above—in theatre with everything ready for Caesarean section.*

2. This form of therapy be conducted only in a hospital equipped for it.

3. Treatment be not delayed until labour begins, and the dreaded 'inevitable haemorrhage' occurs.

Other Forms of Treatment
(mainly historical)

1. *Willett's Forceps*—applied to the fetal scalp can hold the head down into the lower segment, and by applying a weight may keep pressure on the placenta to control the bleeding. Fetal loss—43%. This form of treatment is now used only if the baby be dead.

2. *Bipolar Version and Plugging the Lower Segment with the Half Breech.* Fetal loss, 78% (now only used if the baby be dead or not viable).

Fetal Mortality under the Conservative Régime

Now has been reduced to less than 10%.

Placenta Praevia diagnosed before Bleeding

1. If there be an unusually high presenting part, or an unexplained transverse lie, especially in a primigravida after 36 weeks' gestation, suspect placenta praevia and perform placental localization.
2. If placenta praevia be proved, proceed as though antepartum haemorrhage had occurred (*see above*). However, if a minor degree of placenta praevia be discovered on routine ultrasonography under 34 weeks' gestation, admission could be delayed until 34 weeks: if, then, repeat examination still shows the placenta reaching the lower segment and the head is not already below the placental margin then admission must occur at 34 weeks.

11 Rhesus Factor

ANTIGENS AND ANTIBODIES

Antigens and Immunization

Antigens are substances, usually proteins, which produce a defence mechanism in a subject into which they are injected. This mechanism results in the production of *antibodies* which neutralize the invading antigens. This production of antibodies is known as *immunization.*

Examples

Antigen	*Antibody*
Diphtheria toxin or toxoid	Diphtheria antitoxin
Smallpox vaccine	Smallpox antibodies
Rhesus factor	Anti-rhesus antibodies
These are *acquired* antibodies.	

Natural Antibodies

Also exist, i.e. they are present at birth. These are seen in connexion with the ABO blood group system.

Antigen	*Antibody*
(agglutinogen on the red cells)	(agglutinin in the plasma)
A	α
B	β

It follows that no person with the agglutinogen A on his or her red cells can tolerate α in the plasma: similarly, with B and β. Thus a table can be drawn up of the effect of putting particular cells into the plasma of any other group.

If agglutination occurs we get what is known as a *transfusion reaction.* Cells are destroyed and the products of cell destruction lead to rigors, kidney damage and death.

		$O(AB)$	$\beta(A)$	$\alpha(B)$	$\alpha\beta(O)$
	AB		+	+	+
Cells	A	—		+	+
	B	—	+		+
	O	—	—	—	

+ = agglutination; — = no agglutination.

The Effect of Rhesus Antibodies

The effect of rhesus antibodies on cells containing the Rhesus antigen (or factor) is to cause haemolysis of the red cell with a similar transfusion reaction. These antibodies are therefore called 'haemolysins'. If a person with Rh antibodies, whether produced by previous transfusion or by autoimmunization (q.v.), is transfused with Rh-positive blood, she will get a reaction as serious as that with ABO incompatibility.

Historical Note

In 1940 Landsteiner and Wiener discovered in human red cells an antigen previously known to exist in Rhesus monkeys: they called it, therefore, the 'Rh factor'.

In 1941 Levine and his co-workers found the connexion between the Rh factor and a group of fetal conditions collectively known under the name *erythroblastosis* (*vide infra*).

Incidence of the RH Factor in the Population

Eighty-five per cent of the population possess the factor on their red cells and are called 'Rh-positive'.

Fifteen per cent of the population do not possess the factor on their red cells and are called Rh-negative.

Methods by which Anti-Rh Antibodies are Produced

1. *Transfusion* of Rh-negative patients with Rh-positive blood.

2. *Intramuscular injections of blood,* even as little as 0·05 ml.

3. *Autoimmunization in pregnancy,* where the Rh factor carried on the red cells of the fetus produces antibodies in the mother's plasma. The father must be Rh-positive in order to give the fetus its Rh factor. This mechanism presumes that some fetal red cells pass the placental barrier ('fetomaternal transfusion' or 'transplacental haemorrhage') and give the mother a mis-matched 'transfusion'.

Incidence of Autoimmunization (before the introduction of prophylaxis):

a. Among all births was 1 in 200.

N.B. In 1 in 10 births we have the combination of Rh-negative mother and Rh-positive father. Therefore antibodies only occur in 1 in 20 cases where the appropriate groups are to be found.

b. In Rh-negative women according to birth number:

Birth Number	Incidence
1	Nil
2	1 in 35
3	1 in 21
4	1 in 18
5	1 in 10
6	1 in 7
7	1 in 5

ERYTHROBLASTOSIS OR HAEMOLYTIC DISEASE OF THE NEWBORN

Erythroblastosis is so called because in all conditions grouped under this title the blood contains some immature red cells, known as 'erythroblasts', which are not normally present there. They have been turned out by the bone marrow as an emergency measure to replace the cells lost by the widespread haemolysis. Haemolytic disease of the newborn is now a more generally used term.

Clinical Conditions in Ascending Order of Severity

Haemolytic Anaemia
Immediate, or delayed up to 8 weeks from birth.

Icterus Gravis Neonatorum
1. Anaemia is always present as well as jaundice.
2. In some cases, the basal ganglia of the brain are affected by the pigment, and neurological symptoms occur, e.g. opisthotonos and lethargy. This is called *kernicterus.* Many of those which survive, having shown neurological signs earlier, develop spasticity of the lower limbs or mental deficiency.

Hydrops Fetalis
1. Generalized oedema with fluid in serous cavities.
2. Severe anaemia.
3. Born dead or died shortly after birth.

Macerated Stillbirths
These may result as early as at 26 weeks' gestation. Earlier abortion, however, is never due to rhesus incompatibility.

Differential Diagnosis

1. 'Physiological' jaundice—occurs after 24 hours or even 48 hours from birth.
2. Hydrops fetalis.
a. Syphilis.
b. Diabetic babies.
c. Idiopathic.

Coombs' Test

If incomplete or blocking antibodies are held on the surface of red cells, those cells are doomed, but the presence of the antibodies is not immediately apparent. If, however, the cells are put into contact with anti-human globulin antibodies (prepared in laboratory animals), there will be an antigen–antibody reaction (for the blocking antibodies on the surface of the cells are human globulins) and the cells will haemolyse.

Direct Coombs' Test
This test, performed on the baby's red cells from the cord blood, if *positive,* shows the baby is affected. If *negative,* the baby is safe.

Indirect Coombs' Test
This test is performed on the serum of pregnant women. The serum is put into contact with donor red cells which will absorb the antibodies, if present, on to their surface. If a Coombs' test performed on these cells is now *positive* there were *antibodies in the maternal serum.* This is used as a screening test, for example, on the blood of women attending the antenatal clinic for their first visit.

CDE and cde

The Rhesus is more complex than at first thought. More than six antigens have been described. What was originally called the 'Rh factor' is now designated 'D' and the patients are described as D-positive or D-negative. Erythroblastosis due to antigens other than 'D' can occur, but it is more rare. Antibodies to 'C' 'E', 'c' and 'e' have been identified but not to 'd'. Only anti-C and anti-E antibodies are likely to affect the baby. Such antibodies are more likely to be created by mismatched blood transfusion than autoimmunization.

Treatment

The Blood used for Transfusion should be Rh-negative (as it will not be affected by the antibodies), but *not* the mother's blood, which contains antibodies.

Exchange Transfusion is the treatment of choice when any treatment is required at birth.
1. *Treatment* is given if (i) the cord-blood serum bilirubin exceeds 70 μmol/l (4 mg/100 ml), regardless of the haemoglobin

level, or (ii) the cord-blood haemoglobin falls below 11 g/dl regardless of the serum bilirubin.

2. *Method.* A polythene catheter is inserted along the umbilical vein, and can be used for withdrawing and inserting the blood.

3. *Time after Birth* when the technique is possible is up to 18 hours, but in practice it should be done much earlier.

4. *Quantities* (i) 10–20 ml at a time withdrawn or inserted; (ii) 180 ml/kg of body weight are exchanged (twice the total circulating blood volume), i.e., 27 turns with a 20-ml syringe are required for a 3-kg baby.

5. *Repeat Transfusion* is performed where indicated: the polythene catheter can be left in situ until no longer required.

Simple Transfusion may be required for a case where anaemia develops later. If the baby has a positive Coombs' test it should be followed up for at least 8 weeks with weekly or fortnightly haemoglobin estimations.

1. *Quantity.* 50 ml.

2. *Rate.* Take 20–30 min, i.e. 30 drops/min. Any further blood should be at 10 drops/min.

Premature Delivery of the Fetus by surgical induction or by Caesarean section, in order to offer exchange transfusion before the baby dies or suffers irrevocable damage.

(Premature delivery of all cases where antibodies were present, as practised at one time, was shown by controlled study to produce worse results than inducing no case at all.)

To select the appropriate cases and the optimum time for premature delivery the following methods are available:

1. *Previous History*

DISADVANTAGE. No help when the first manifestation is a fatal one.

PRACTICAL APPLICATION

a. Where a baby has been lost in a previous

pregnancy delivery of the baby at a safe period of gestation may produce a successful outcome. However, the hazard of prematurity has to be weighed against any virtue that may accrue from premature delivery.

b. When there is a history of a previous severe manifestation amniocentesis may give a guide when to deliver the baby (*see below*).

2. *Estimation of Antibody Levels in Maternal Serum*

DISADVANTAGES

a. The correlation between antibody level and effect in the baby is a very loose one, so that this method gives only a rough guide to prognosis.

b. Antibodies once present do not recede, so that estimation is only of help before dangerous levels are reached; thereafter it gives no guidance as to when to deliver the baby, e.g. if a level of 64 i.u./ml is found at the outset of the pregnancy.

LEVELS. These can be interpreted as follows:

International units per ml	Titre	Degree of involvement
0–16	1 in 20	Mild or unaffected
17–32	1 in 40	Moderate
33–64 and over	1 in 80 and over	Severe

PRACTICAL APPLICATION. Antibody levels can be estimated routinely at 28 and 34 weeks' gestation. If the level does not indicate a significant involvement serial estimations at fortnightly intervals can be studied. If the level exceeds 16 i.u./ml amniocentesis should be performed.

3. *Amniocentesis and Estimation of Bilirubin in the Liquor Spectroscopically*

PRACTICAL APPLICATION. 5–10 ml of liquor are taken when the previous history or the antibody level indicates it.

The optical density graph is studied and the degree of fetal involvement is related to the size of the 'bulge' at a wavelength of 450 nm.

The height of this 'bulge' above the base line is referred to as the 'optical density'. The value of this is plotted on Liley's prediction charts, according to the period of gestation, and the anticipated degree of fetal involvement is read off.

a. Delivery is considered, taking this into account along with the previous history and the period of gestation, e.g. 35 weeks or even less for severe cases, 38 weeks for mild and moderate cases.

b. If there has been a previous severe manifestation and the husband is heterozygous, amniocentesis will make it possible to distinguish between an Rh-negative baby which will not be affected and an Rh-positive one which is in severe danger, thereby avoiding unnecessary premature delivery of an unaffected baby.

Intra-uterine Fetal Transfusion

1. *Peritoneal*

a. Principal. Red cells are absorbed as such from the fetal peritoneum. This does not occur in adults.

b. Choice of Case. Where there is virtually no chance of survival of the baby by induction as judged by the previous history, the husband being homozygous, or, if heterozygous, amniocentesis shows the baby to be affected.

c. Time for Transfusion. Earlier than the previous intra-uterine deaths. The transferred blood cells will survive for about 3 weeks.

d. Technique

　i. The baby's position is ascertained by X-ray examination.

　ii. Under local anaesthesia a needle is introduced into the fetal abdominal cavity.

　iii. A polythene catheter is introduced into the abdominal cavity and 2 ml of urografin are injected. X-ray of the fetus will show the contrast medium outlining the abdominal cavity.

iv. 100 ml of packed red cells are injected in 30 min.

v. The catheter is withdrawn.

vi. After delivery, the cord blood is estimated for the relative proportions of donor and fetal blood, and it is found that the blood may be predominantly that of the donor.

2. *Into Umbilical Artery via the Fetoscope.* Is now possible in some centres and may save babies that would have no chance of survival by any other technique.

Plasmapheresis

Maternal blood is withdrawn, the cells are separated from the plasma, resuspended in donor plasma free of anti-D antibody and then returned to the pregnant woman; it is a continuous process.

By doing this at frequent intervals intra-uterine transfusion may be avoided.

Prevention of Autoim-munization

There is evidence that the most usual time for fetal red cells to cross the placental barrier into the maternal circulation, thereby creating antibodies, is during labour, but such cells will only survive if there is compatibility between them and the maternal plasma. Where they do survive, they can be detected by a slide technique, which distinguishes the fetal haemoglobin in these cells from that found in the adult cells of the mother (the Kleihauer test).

These fetal cells will be D-positive and, if potent anti-D serum is given after delivery in these cases, the invading cells will be destroyed and antibody formation prevented. *An injection of potent anti-D gammaglobulin is given within 72 hours to all D-negative women, who have not already acquired anti-D antibodies, having: (i) been delivered of a D-positive baby or (ii) had a termination of pregnancy without sterilization.*

Prognosis

1. Not all babies born in the presence of antibodies discovered in pregnancy will require treatment after birth.

2. Not all babies with a positive Coombs' test will require treatment.

3. Cases occurring for the first time in the second pregnancy tend to be more severe than those occurring in subsequent pregnancies.

4. Cases following immunization by transfusion tend to be more severe than those following auto-immunization.

5. Babies showing neurological signs with jaundice are likely to be abnormal if they survive.

6. Future pregnancies when antibodies are present:

a. If the manifestation occurs at all, it will be as severe the next time, if not more so.

b. The husband's Rh group may be of assistance:

i. If he be Rh-negative (dd)—the baby will escape.

ii. If he be heterozygous positive (Dd)—the baby has a 50% chance of escaping.

iii. If he be homozygous positive (DD)—the baby will be affected.

Application in Antenatal Care

1. All patients are tested at the first visit to the clinic for their Rh group.

2. Re-testing for antibodies is required in the following cases at 28 *and* 34 *weeks:*

a. All Rh-negative patients in their second or subsequent pregnancy.

b. All cases with a history of a previous transfusion.

c. All cases with a history of intramuscular injections of blood.

d. All cases with a history of previous unexplained stillbirth.

3. If the local centre can cope with the work it is desirable to test the *husbands* of all Rh-negative women. If the husband is Rh-negative too, no further testing of the mother need be done in this or any future pregnancy by that husband.

4. *Advice needs to be given to Rh-negative mothers* who are anxious on the following lines:

a. The 'Rh-negative' merely means a certain type of blood shared by 15% of people.

b. In the first pregnancy, the baby will be quite healthy (assuming no history of transfusion).

c. Future babies should be protected from Rhesus disease by the injection given, where required, after this and subsequent deliveries.

d. Even if treatment has to be given, in almost all cases it is successful in producing a healthy baby.

e. If the husband is tested and is shown to be Rh-negative, there is no fear of the baby being affected.

APPLICATION OF THE RHESUS FACTOR TO TRANSFUSION

1. No woman under menopausal age must ever be given Rh-positive blood if she be Rh-negative; it may prevent her ever having a live baby.

2. If the Rh group is unknown and cannot be found quickly enough, Rh-negative blood must be given.

3. It is preferable never to give Rh-positive blood to an Rh-negative person of any sex or any age. It must certainly not be done if there has been a previous transfusion.

HYPERBILIRUBINAEMIA

Sometimes the so-called 'physiological jaundice' can reach levels which can be dangerous to the baby by the production of kernicterus: this danger is greatest in premature babies. In such cases if the serum bilirubin should reach or exceed 340 μmol/l (20 mg/100 ml) exchange transfusion is performed.

12 Polyhydramnios

DEFINITION

An excess of liquor amnii.
An amount in excess of 2 litres may be taken as the arbitrary standard of abnormality, but the diagnosis is really made clinically (*see below*).

CAUSES

Fetal

1. Multiple pregnancy (reason unknown).
2. Abnormality.

Types. Mainly anencephaly (48 out of 74 abnormal babies—Macafee).

Causal Hypotheses
a. The abnormal fetus does not swallow properly (*see* 'Circulation of Amniotic Fluid').
b. In high alimentary obstruction, e.g. duodenal atresia, the gut surface for absorption is much reduced.
c. Cases with an open subarachnoid space may contribute C.S.F. to the amniotic fluid, increasing its bulk.

Incidence of Abnormality and its Detection by X-rays (Macafee C. H. G. (1950) *J. Obstet. Gynaecol. Br.Emp.,* **57,** 171)

a. X-rays showed
   abnormality   54 cases
b. Further
   abnormalities
   found after
   birth   20 cases 74 abnormal cases
c. Normal infants   58 normal cases

          Total   132

Therefore:
a. In just under half the cases of polyhydramnios the baby will be normal.
b. In one-quarter of cases with a normal radiograph the baby will still be abnormal.

3. Hydrops fetalis.

Maternal
1. Diabetes mellitus.
2. Congestive heart failure.

Unknown Causes

SYMPTOMS

1. Dyspnoea (if abdomen is greatly distended).
2. Abdominal pain (if onset is acute or subacute).
3. Vomiting (in acute cases).

SIGNS

1. Tense uterus—fetal parts difficult to palpate, but are usually ballotable to some extent.
2. Fluid thrill.

3. Abnormal presentation, and in any case presenting part is high.
4. Abdomen very large—exceeds 1 metre at full term (in practice not a helpful sign as so much depends on the degree of obesity).
5. Fetal heart may be difficult to hear but is usually present.
N.B.   *True acute polyhydramnios* is very rare. It usually occurs early in pregnancy and is associated with uni-ovular twins. The swelling comes on very rapidly and there is severe pain and vomiting.

DANGERS

1. Malpresentation.
2. Prolapsed cord.
3. Premature rupture of membranes.
4. Postpartum haemorrhage.
N.B.   It has been taught that prolonged labour is associated with polyhydramnios, but this has been denied by Jeffcoate.

TREATMENT

1. If abnormal on X-ray examination, admit to hospital:
a. Rupture the forewaters when 36 weeks or over (attempts to induce labour by surgical means earlier may fail and intra-uterine sepsis may develop which would be a disaster), or
b. Cause the uterus to empty itself by means of either (i) intra-amniotic prostaglandin, or (ii) intravenous prostaglandin.
2. If normal on X-ray examination:
a. Await spontaneous onset of labour unless there is great discomfort.
b. If severe, admit to hospital to await labour (danger of abnormal lie and prolapse of cord). If the discomfort is great and the baby is too premature for surgical induction of labour, tapping of the amniotic cavity per abdomen

with very gradual release of the fluid may relieve the symptoms without starting labour: the polyhydramnios does not necessarily re-form. This procedure is very seldom justified.

c. Vaginal examination immediately the membranes rupture.

d. Anticipate postpartum haemorrhage by i.v. ergometrine with the anterior shoulder.

N.B.   The really acute form may need termination of the pregnancy.

3. After delivery in such cases be aware of the possibility of oesophageal atresia or other gastro-intestinal obstruction requiring urgent surgery. Excessive 'drooling', or spluttering and cyanosis with administration of sterile water by mouth should draw attention to this danger.

If oesophageal atresia is suspected pass an oesophageal tube into the upper part of the oesophagus and keep it empty by aspiration until the baby is ready for surgery. This will protect the baby's lungs.

13 | **Fetal Abnormality**

AETIOLOGY

(Unknown in many cases)

Infections in Early Pregnancy

The **rubella virus** is the only infection that has been implicated definitely as a significant cause of congenital deformities (other than congenital syphilis).

Types of Abnormality

Congenital heart disease	4·7%	⎫ Incidence in women
Cataract	4·7%	with rubella during first 12 weeks of
Deafness	3·0%	⎭ pregnancy
Mental deficiency		

Period of Gestation when rubella produces a significant effect is in the first 12 weeks only (with a very small effect between 12 and 16 weeks).

Incidence of Abnormality (Reports on Public Health and Medical Subjects, No. 101).

	Rubella up to 12 Weeks	Controls
Abortions (%)	5·0	2·4
Stillbirths (%)	4·5	2·4
Children dying under 2 years (%)	6·9	2·4
Major malformations in children surviving to 2 years (%)	13·0	2·3

Some milder cases of deafness, but no other abnormality, were detected in children between the ages of 3 and 5 years, but in only a small proportion of these was deafness a severe handicap.

Women in the first 16 weeks of pregnancy who have been contacts with a case of suggested rubella.

1. Gammaglobulin 750 mg i.m. should be given as soon as possible though its effectiveness is open to doubt. If the immunological state of the mother can be ascertained quickly this should be done first.

2. Blood is taken for rubella antibody tests:

If the titre is high shortly after the contact the pregnant woman is immune and the baby is safe.

If the titre is low on the first test and 3–4 weeks later it rises, with or without the overt signs of rubella, the baby is at risk and termination of pregnancy should be offered.

If the titre is high when the first test is at least 4 weeks after the contact it is difficult to tell whether there has been subclinical infection or not, but the chances are that the antibodies are long-standing and termination would not be indicated.

Women in the first 16 weeks of pregnancy with clinical signs resembling rubella.

a. If the antibody titre is low and remains so it is not rubella and the baby is safe.

b. If the antibody titre rises over a 3-week observation period, termination should be offered.

c. If the first test is at least 3 weeks after onset of the rash and shows a high titre, rubella cannot be excluded and termination must be considered.

Prophylaxis. Women who on blood testing show a low rubella antibody titre can be immunized but:

1. The vaccine, which consists of live virus, may be as dangerous to a fetus as a rubella infection in the mother. Thus, it must be

absolutely certain that the woman is not pregnant before giving the injection. Immediately after delivery is probably the safest time. If a mistake is made termination must be considered.
2. There is doubt as to how long the effect of immunization lasts.

Genetic Factors

(*see* Antenatal Diagnosis of Fetal Abnormalities)
1. Chromosomal abnormalities, e.g. trisomy 21 (Down's syndrome, Mongolism).
2. Metabolic disorders, e.g. Tay-Sachs disease, congenital adrenal hyperplasia, phenylketonuria, hypothyroidism—and many others.
3. X-linked recessives, e.g. haemophilia, Duchenne's muscular dystrophy.
4. Neural tube defects, e.g. anencephaly, spina bifida, hydrocephaly.
5. Haemoglobinopathies, e.g. sickle-cell disease, thalassaemia.
6. Autosomal dominants, e.g. achondroplasia, Huntington's chorea.
7. Autosomal recessives, e.g. cystic fibrosis.

Drugs

1. *Thalidomide* in the early weeks of pregnancy produced limb deformities. This is the only known case of major deformities produced by a drug in widespread use, but it has caused everybody to be on the alert for any new drug which may result in similar disaster.
2. *Tetracycline* given after the 16th week of pregnancy may produce colour changes, (e.g. yellow fluorescence), caries and enamel hypoplasia in the infant's teeth. (It may also predispose to liver damage in the mother when given in the last trimester of pregnancy.)
3. *Warfarin and other oral anticoagulants* (in first trimester). Chondroplasia punctata; nasal hypoplasia; small for dates; brachydactylia, etc.

4. *Anti-epileptic drugs.* Especially phenytoin and phenobarbitone. (Sodium valproate appears to be the drug of choice but it can cause thrombocytopenia.) The risks are small and of a minor nature.

5. *Alcohol*—in heavy drinkers. Growth retardation and abnormal facial features.

6. *Co-trimoxazole*—a possible effect.

7. *Certain progestogens,* e.g. norethisterone. Virilization in female fetuses.

8. *Cytotoxic drugs.* Especially alkylating agents and methotrexate. High risk of teratogenesis.

9. *Non-steroidal anti-inflammatory agents* e.g. aspirin; indomethacin. Cause closure of ductus arteriosus in utero and possibly persistent pulmonary hypertension in the neonate. Avoid in later weeks of pregnancy.

10. *Podophyllum resin*—used over wide areas. Fetal death and teratogenesis.

N.B. With many new drugs the manufacturers warn that caution must be used when using the drugs in pregnancy—a commendable cautiousness, though it may be tinged by the fear of litigation. In such cases the clinician has to weigh the advantages of the drug against the possible, though unproven, risks.

Radiation

Evidence of its Importance

1. Irradiation of *Drosophila* flies produced mutations in succeeding generations.

2. Irradiation of mammal embryos at a period of gestation, corresponding to the 2nd to the 6th week of human pregnancy, when organs are in the process of development, may lead to abnormalities.

3. The effect of exposing pregnant women to severe dosage of radiation at Nagasaki led to more than half the children being stillborn, dying in the neonatal period, or becoming mentally retarded.

4. Diagnostic radiography in the antenatal period carries a small but significant increase in the incidence of leukaemia and cancer in childhood.

Conclusion
Exposure to radiation should at all times be kept to a minimum, especially in pregnant women. Pelvic radiation in fertile women should be avoided in the 2 weeks before the period whenever possible. However, where information of direct clinical use can be obtained, carefully controlled radiography need not be withheld.

ASSOCIATED FACTORS

1. Polyhydramnios (q.v.).
2. Diabetes mellitus—incidence is 6·3% and it is usually accompanied by polyhydramnios.

TYPES OF ABNORMALITY

Many malformations lead to abortion and are never diagnosed. There is an immense variety of abnormalities to be found in babies at term, but the following are the most important.

Abnormalities causing Difficulty in Labour

Hydrocephalus
Pathology
1. There is an abnormally large head due to distension of the cerebral ventricles caused by an obstruction to the flow and absorption of cerebrospinal fluid.
2. The cranial sutures and fontanelles are very wide.
3. There is no special tendency to polyhydramnios.
Importance. The large head cannot pass the brim, so labour will become obstructed. It is, however, a rare condition.
Diagnosis
1. *In Pregnancy:*
a. Large head felt on abdominal palpation.
b. Overlap despite a normal pelvis.

2. *In Labour:*
a. Failure of head to engage despite an adequate pelvis.
b. Wide sutures felt on vaginal examination.
c. Head sticks at the brim when delivering a breech; there will often be a lumbar spina bifida as well.
N.B. Ultimate diagnosis rests on: (1) Palpation of wide sutures; (2) X-ray findings, including cephalometry; (3) Ultrasonography showing enlarged ventricles.
Treatment. Perforation of the head during labour, after which delivery should be easy.

Fetal Tumours may be large enough to obstruct delivery. They are rare.
Examples
1. Teratoma in the cervical or sacral region.
2. Abdominal swelling:
a. Polycystic kidneys.
b. Ascites.

Conjoined Twins may be joined in many different ways. Delivery will usually be by Caesarean section or by destructive procedures per vaginam. Occasionally spontaneous delivery occurs.

Abnormalities of Importance after Delivery

A few only are mentioned.

Incompatible with Continued Life, even if Born Alive
1. Anencephaly.
2. Severe forms of spina bifida.

Often Amenable to Operative Treatment
1. Hare lip and cleft palate.
2. Imperforate anus.
3. Duodenal diaphragm.
4. Milder forms of spina bifida and hydrocephaly.
5. Accessory digits and auricles.
N.B. Bony abnormalities may have been detected before delivery, a radiograph having been taken for hydramnios. Soft-tissue abnormalities cannot be detected till after delivery.

Fetal Death in Utero

DIAGNOSIS (*see also* Chapter 15)

Clinically

1. The uterus fails to grow in size or even shrinks while under observation for a month or even two. A single observation may be misleading as the dates may be wrong.
2. *a.* No fetal heart is heard even with an ultrasound fetal heart detector.
b. The fetal heart can no longer be heard when it has been heard previously.

Ultra-sonography

1. Fetal heart beat not seen.
2. No fetal movements seen.
3. Fetus fails to grow over a period of 2 weeks or more.

X-ray confirmation

This is sometimes possible, but no help can be given until the fetus has been dead for some time.
1. Spalding's sign (overlap and angulation of skull bones).
2. The ball sign (the toneless fetus is wrapped up like a ball).

MANAGEMENT

1. Under 12 weeks. Evacuation of the uterus in one stage is possible.
2. Over 12 weeks.
a. An oxytocin drip may be tried but it often fails.
b. Prostaglandins by i.v. route are usually successful. Oxytocin can be given at the same time to speed things up.
N.B. It is usually held that to rupture the membranes when the fetus is dead may be dangerous, but some dissent from this view.

CLOTTING DEFECT

Clotting defect causing postpartum haemorrhage may occur after delivery when the fetus has been dead for 3 weeks or more.

MATERNITY GRANT

Maternity grant is payable if the 28th week was reached before the uterus was emptied regardless of the size of the fetus.

DEFINITION

Expulsion of the uterine contents under the 28th week of gestation.

COMMONEST TIME FOR ABORTION

This is at the 12th week.

1. The villi have not yet invaded deeply.

2. There is a period of instability, with a drop in progesterone output, when the corpus luteum is regressing and the placenta may not yet have taken over the function of progesterone production.

3. Even in pregnancy the pituitary gland is probably undergoing its cyclic activity, giving an impulse to the uterus once a month. Such an impulse, coming at the time of instability, may account for the frequency of abortion at the time when the third missed period would have arrived.

143

THREATENED AND INEVITABLE ABORTION

Clinical Presentation

	Threatened	Inevitable
1. —		Part of the ovum extruded.
2. *Pain*	Absent or infrequent.	Regular contractions.
3. *Bleeding*	Slight or moderate.	Slight, moderate or severe.
4. *Cervix*	Closed.	Dilatation beginning.
5. *Ultra-sonography*	Fetal heart beat is seen.	Fetal heart beat not seen.

Treatment

Threatened

1. Rest and sedation.

2. Allow up when bleeding has ceased for some days.

Inevitable

1. Blood transfusion if required.

2. Ergometrine 0·25 mg i.v. and 0·25 mg i.m., or 0·5 mg i.m., to control bleeding.

3. *a.* Under 12 weeks—immediate evacuation of the uterus.
   b. Over 12 weeks—*see* Chapter 14, 'Fetal Death in Utero'.

INCOMPLETE ABORTION

Part of the ovum left in the uterus can cause severe bleeding.
Ultrasonography will show retained products of conception if present (if none are seen the patient can be spared operation).

Treatment

As under 'Inevitable' abortion, emptying the uterus in theatre at once.

SEPTIC ABORTION

Clinically

As for 'Inevitable' or 'Incomplete' abortion, and in addition:
1. General signs of sepsis.
2. Lower abdominal pain.
3. Offensive bloodstained discharge.

Treatment

1. Antibiotics, after taking a vaginal swab.
2. Postpone evacuation of the uterus for at least 24 hours, and maybe until the temperature has been settled for several days, unless bleeding demands instant action.

MISSED ABORTION

Missed abortion is fetal death in utero, the fetus having been completely retained. (*See* Chapter 14, 'Fetal Death in Utero'.)

COMPLICATIONS OF ALL FORMS

Irreversible Shock

Anuria

(Bilateral renal cortical necrosis or lower nephron nephrosis.) Most likely after abortion complicated by shock or sepsis (cf. Eclampsia and Accidental Haemorrhage).

Sepsis

Sepsis leading to (i) Death; or (ii) Infertility due to tubal damage.

Pituitary Necrosis

Pituitary necrosis may occur as a remote effect, where there has been severe haemorrhage.

Clinically

1. *Sheehan's Disease*

a. Amenorrhoea.

b. Loss of axillary and pubic hair.

c. Hypoglycaemia.

d. Feels cold easily.

2. *Simmonds' Disease* (more rare). Premature senility.

CAUSES OF HABITUAL ABORTION

N.B. A case is not regarded as habitual until after three previous abortions. Fewer than this could so easily be due to chance.

Maternal Causes

(Also lead to premature labour)

Local

a. Fibroids.

b. Hypoplasia of the uterus.

c. Double uterus.

d. Deep cervical laceration.

e. Amputation of cervix.

f. Incompetent internal cervical os:
  Period of gestation   16 weeks or over.
  Diagnosis   History of recurrent expulsion of a fresh fetus: often the membranes will rupture before contractions begin. There is also, commonly, a history of a previous therapeutic abortion per vaginam.
  Treatment: Shirodkar operation at 14 weeks. This is the insertion of a non-absorbable suture around the cervix at the level of the internal os. It is removed at 38 weeks and spontaneous labour is allowed to occur.

General

a. Syphilis (only after 20th week).

b. Nephritis.

c. Essential hypertension.

d. Diabetes mellitus.

e. Rhesus factor (only after 26th week).

Fetal Abnormality	Recurrent. There is a high incidence of chromosomal abnormalities in aborted fetusus. Perform chromosomal studies on parents and on the fetus, if available.
Idiopathic	These include cases presumed to be due to hormonal disturbance. The majority of cases fall into this group, i.e. there is no obvious cause.

Treatment. There is evidence that even if no treatment be given 80% of cases in this group, having had three or more previous abortions, will nevertheless go to term—the outcome one would expect in any normal pregnancy (Bevis, D. C. A. (1951) *Lancet,* Aug. 4, 207). Notwithstanding, most gynaecologists, including the author, feel a need, however illogical, to offer therapy with a non-virilizing oral progestogen, e.g. Medroxyprogesterone 5 mg tds, until well past the period of gestation of the most advanced previous fetal death. Selection of cases for this treatment may be by:
1. Vaginal smear (a high proportion of cornified cells indicates progesterone deficiency).
2. Cervical smear ('Ferning', i.e. the production of crystals in the dried mucus on a slide, suggests progesterone deficiency).

HYDATIDIFORM MOLE

Cause	Unknown
Pathology	**1.** *a.* The chorionic villi become oedematous and form vesicles a few millimetres in diameter. *b.* As a rule no fetus is seen but there can be partial degeneration of an abortion placenta and then the fetus may be present. **2.** High output of chorionic gonadotrophin

from the markedly hypertrophied trophoblast.
3. Both ovaries are markedly enlarged by the presence of multiple theca-lutein cysts due to chorionic gonadotrophin stimulation.
4. There is about a 10% incidence of choriocarcinoma following hydatidiform mole.

Clinical Presentation

1. *a.* Like abortion, i.e. *amenorrhoea* followed by *bleeding.*
b. The uterus may be: (i) larger than the dates indicate if actively growing; (ii) smaller than the dates if not actively growing; (iii) in agreement with the dates.
c. The enlarged ovaries may be palpable.
2. The mole may be *extruded,* wholly or partially: the vesicles are diagnostic.
3. There may be: *a. Pre-eclampsia*—much earlier in pregnancy than usual.
b. Hyperemesis gravidarum—severe.

Investigation

1. *Ultrasonography* is diagnostic: the vesicle surface forms an interface which is displayed by ultrasound. No other investigation is necessary.
2. *a.* Estimation of urinary *chorionic gonadotrophin* by radioimmune assay gives levels higher than the top limit of normal for the period of gestation.
b. Pregnancy test positive in dilution of 1 in 100 is highly suspicious.
N.B. These hormonal effects are only positive in an actively growing mole—they are, however, often negative.

Treatment

1. *Evacuation of the uterus,* whatever its size, preferably by the suction evacuator. Give 0·5 mg of ergometrine i.v. immediately before operating.
2. *Abdominal hysterectomy* may be the treatment of choice if no further children are required—it obviates the risk of subsequent choriocarcinoma.

3. The enlarged *ovaries* will subside and do not require removal.

4. A *routine D and C* is performed 7 days later to remove any residual material which might become malignant.

Follow-up

Follow-up to detect the development of choriocarcinoma.

It is so eminently treatable that failure to detect it is a major calamity.

1. *a.* Follow-up is preferably for 2 years although 1 year is acceptable if the patient is anxious to get pregnant again as soon as possible.

b. Contraception must be employed as a pregnancy vitiates the result. There is divided opinion as to whether the oral contraceptive pill should be employed.

2. Monthly 24-hour specimens of urine are collected and an aliquot is sent for estimation of the chorionic gonadotrophin. This returns to normal within 4 weeks of the evacuation of a mole and should remain thus in the absence of choriocarcinoma or a new pregnancy.

3. *Treatment of choriocarcinoma* is very successful by chemotherapy, notably by methotrexate. Operation is not usually necessary.

N.B. Follow-up and treatment can be undertaken by specially designated centres in the UK, e.g. at the Jessop Hospital, Sheffield; if the centre is notified the case will be managed from there, the original clinician being notified of all results.

Part 2
Labour and the Puerperium

Physiology of Labour

DEFINITION OF LABOUR

The process by which a viable fetus, together with its placenta, umbilical cord, membranes and liquor amnii, is expelled or removed from the mother's body.

CAUSE OF ONSET OF LABOUR

This is unknown, but we observe an increasing irritability of uterus towards term. We do not know with certainty why this should be, nor can we explain with confidence the remarkable phenomenon of labour occurring in most cases so near to the calculated date. The following factors may be considered:

Hormonal

1. There is a marked drop in progesterone secretion just before labour. Progesterone is believed to be necessary for the continuation of pregnancy.

2. There is an increase of 'free' oestrogen just before labour, i.e. it is being released from its combined form which is inert. Oestrogen is believed to increase the responsiveness of uterine muscle to normal circulating amounts of oxytocin.

3. The pituitary is believed to be maintaining its cyclic activity, even during pregnancy, and with successive monthly impulse there is a tendency for the uterus to empty itself. At the tenth cycle after conception the uterus is 'ripe' for that particular impulse to take effect, and labour occurs. This may also account for the tendency for abortion to occur at the 12th week, i.e. the third cycle, a temporary fall in progesterone output at the time rendering the uterus susceptible.

Increased Uterine Distension	**1.** Stretching muscle fibres increases their power of contraction. **2.** Interference with the uterine and placental circulation may produce a reduction in placental hormonal output.
Pressure of the Fetus on the Lower Uterine Segment	Stimulating the upper segment to contract (bipolarity).

STAGES OF LABOUR

First Stage	Dilatation of the cervix.
Second Stage	From full dilatation to complete expulsion of the fetus.
Third Stage	Separation and expulsion of the placenta and membranes.

Upper Limit of Normal Duration of Labour

	Primigravidae	*Multigravidae*
First stage	12 hours	9 hours
Second stage	1 hour	¾ hour
Third stage	½ hour	½ hour

The figures for the first stage of labour have little practical significance; they can be exceeded with impunity if there is no maternal or fetal distress. The important factor is whether there is continued dilatation of cervix over a period of observation (*see* Inefficient uterine action, p. 221).

FACTORS IN LABOUR

Powers

Primary Powers, *i.e.* **the Uterine Musculature**
1. *Upper and Lower Uterine Segments*
a. Development. Arise during the *latter half of pregnancy* but the lower segment is more clearly distinguished in labour. At full term it is about 8 cm wide.

Upper segment arises from the *corpus uteri.*

Lower segment arises from the *isthmus uteri* and the *cervix.* The main expansion is in the isthmus, the cervical part not altering much in length from the beginning of pregnancy to the end of labour.

The *physiological retraction ring* separates the two segments, it being the thickened lower limit of the upper segment. It represents the *anatomical internal os* of the non-pregnant uterus. When exaggerated, as in obstructed labour, it is known as the *pathological retraction ring* or *Bandl's ring.* (Neither of these should be confused with a *contraction or constriction ring* which is a localized spasm of a circle of uterine muscle occurring in a certain type of abnormal uterine action.)
b. Muscle Fibres
Upper Segment: Outer longitudinal. Middle interlacing (the thickest and most important). Inner circular.

Lower Segment: Mainly longitudinal and thin, the structure being largely fibrous.

c. Functions

Upper Segment: Contraction and *relaxation,* as with ordinary muscle. *Retraction,* a special property of uterine muscle. During this the upper segment gets shorter but thicker.

Lower Segment: Mainly passive, being stretched by the upper segment in normal labour. Thus it becomes wider but thinner.

d. Co-ordination of the Two Segments in Action: For the uterus to expel its contents the upper segment must contract strongly and the lower segment remain passive. Failure to achieve this 'Fundal Dominance' means that labour does not progress, e.g.

i. Contractions of *late pregnancy* and of *false labour.*

ii. *Incoordinate uterine action* in prolonged labour. In the last mentioned condition the intra-uterine pressure may reach or exceed that found in normal labour, e.g. approximately 45 mmHg, but yet the cervix does not dilate.

2. *Control of Uterine Action*

a. Inherent Contractibility of Uterine Muscle. Even isolated strips of uterine muscle show rhythmical contraction in a saline bath. This property is the main cause of the uterine activity in menstruation and labour. The method by which upper and lower segment are co-ordinated is not understood.

The uterine action, however, may be modified as follows.

b. Nervous Control by the sympathetic (and perhaps the parasympathetic) nervous system.

The anatomical and physiological extent of this control is still disputed.

The uterus can act perfectly well cut off from all nerve connections.

Emotion, e.g. fear, can affect labour, but whether by a nerve or endocrine route is not known.

c. Hormonal Control. Oxytocin stimulates the uterus, but there is no evidence that its output rises during labour.

Free oestrogens sensitize the uterus to oxytocin: this may be a factor in labour.

Secondary Powers, *i.e.* the Mother's Voluntary Expulsive Efforts

1. *Mechanism*

The intra-abdominal cavity can be regarded as a box with an opening, i.e. the pelvic cavity. The remaining walls are:

a. The maternal spine—rigid.

b. The diaphragm—made rigid by filling the chest with air and holding it so by closing the glottis.

c. The muscles of the anterior and lateral abdominal walls.

As the muscles contract, the room in the abdominal cavity is reduced, the remaining walls being rigid, so the fetus must escape by the only route available, viz. the birth canal.

2. *The Efficiency is Reduced by:*

a. Failure to keep the glottis closed (e.g. grunting or crying out) which allows the diaphram to rise.

b. Failure to draw the abdominal wall in, blowing it out instead.

3. *Control of the Secondary Powers*

Although depending upon the action of *voluntary muscles,* the expulsive effort is called into play *involuntarily* by the pressure of the presenting part on the pelvic floor (cf. the expulsive urge which accompanies a loaded rectum).

Actions of the Powers

1. *Take-up and Dilatation of the Cervix by the Primary Powers* (*Figs.* 11, 12)

a. Take-up means pulling the cervix into line with the rest of the lower segment.

b. In the *primipara* take-up precedes dilatation, the internal os opening first, so that dilatation begins with the external os. In the *multipara* take up and dilatation occur

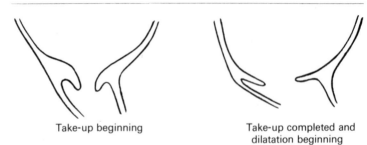

Take-up beginning

Take-up completed and
dilatation beginning

Fig. 11. Take-up and dilatation of the cervix in a
primipara.

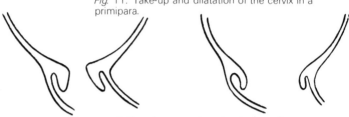

Take-up and dilatation occurring simultaneously.

Fig. 12. Take-up and dilatation of the cervix in a
multipara.

simultaneously, dilatation beginning with the
internal os.

c. The mechanism of this process is the pull
exerted on the lower segment by the retracting
upper segment. It is assisted by downward
thrust of the presenting part or the bag of
forewaters, but it will occur even if neither is
pressing on the cervix. The importance of the
bag of forewaters has been exaggerated: if
anything, the uterus behaves more efficiently if
the membranes are ruptured (but there are
disadvantages of ruptured membranes which
may counterbalance this).

2. *Expulsion of the Uterine Contents*
Expulsion occurs, after full dilatation, by the
primary powers. The upper segment continues
to retract and so the overall length of the
uterus grows less. It is therefore stripping itself
upwards over the fetal ovoid, which is the
same thing as expelling the fetus from its cavity.

3. *Descent of the Fetus*
a. Stages: It may occur in the latter weeks of pregnancy, as well as in the first and second stage of labour.

It may, on the other hand, not occur till the second stage, and after the membranes have ruptured (chiefly in multiparae).

b. Mechanism:

PRIMARY POWERS

The uterine moorings are: (a) The parametrium. (*b*) The layer of fascia running from the uterus down over the vagina. (*c*) The round ligaments (least important).

The *retracting upper segment,* by shortening itself, must drive the fetus down, for the whole uterus cannot rise up on account of its moorings. However, these moorings may be slack in multiparae having been stretched at previous labour: thus, they may not become tense enough to anchor the uterus until much retraction has taken place, perhaps not until the second stage has been reached.

SECONDARY POWERS

These only play a part in the second stage and their mode of action is given above.

4. *Separation of the Placenta in the Third Stage by the Primary Powers*
a. The retraction of the upper segment continues after expulsion of the fetus to a marked degree. The inelastic placenta cannot follow this so it must separate.
b. Retroplacental blood clot may help the separation.

5. *Expulsion of the Placenta in the Third Stage by Primary and Secondary Powers*
a. Expulsion from the uterus by the primary powers.
b. Expulsion from the vagina by the secondary powers. A helping hand may be required.
⎫
⎬ As for the fetus
⎭

6. *Control of Haemorrhage in the Third Stage by the 'Living Ligature Action' of the Primary Powers*

Effect of the Primary Powers on the Mother

Pain is produced with each contraction. This may be due to:

1. *Via Autonomic Sensory Nerves*
Uterine ischaemia—a referred pain as the force of the contractions rises above the systolic blood pressure and so cuts off the flow of blood to the uterine muscle.

2. *Via Somatic Sensory Nerves*
a. Pressure on the pelvic floor and its surroundings.
b. Traction on the uterine moorings.

Effect of the Powers on the Fetus

Slowing of the Fetal Heart rate is often heard at the height of a contraction. It may be due to:

a. Compression of the fetal head, or
b. The temporary cutting off of, or reduction in, the blood flow to the placenta due to a mild application of the 'living ligature' function of the myometrium.

This is really a temporary distress and were it not that the uterine action is intermittent, giving time for recovery, the fetus could hardly survive labour.

Passages

Hard Passages, *i.e.* the Pelvis

1. *True and False Pelvis*
The former is the deep basin below the pelvic brim. The latter is the space embraced by the blades of the ilium.

2. *Planes of the Pelvis*

a. Brim
TRACED FROM BEFORE BACKWARDS
Symphysis pubis.
Iliopectineal line.
Promontory of the sacrum.
INCLINATION OF THE BRIM
Sixty degrees to the horizontal when erect.
Thirty degrees to the horizontal when supine.
N.B. When erect the anterior superior iliac spine is vertically over the symphysis pubis.

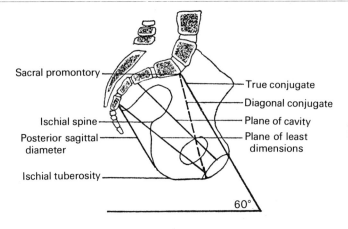

Fig. 13. Diameters of the pelvis in the sagittal plane.

DIAMETERS (*Fig.* 13)
i. ANTEROPOSTERIOR. From the back of the top of the symphysis pubis to the promontory of the sacrum. Also known as: (*a*) *True conjugate;* or (*b*) *Conjugata vera;* or (*c*) *Internal conjugate.*
N.B.   If there be a false promontory at a lower level, a diameter from the back of the symphysis to this point may be less than the true conjugate. This is then called the *obstetrical conjugate.*
ii. TRANSVERSE. The widest diameter across the brim.
N.B.   An *obstetrical transverse diameter of the brim* is described, measured across the brim at a point midway between front and back. In an ideal pelvis the two are identical. In a shield-shaped pelvis where the widest diameter is far back the obstetrical transverse diameter may be considerably less.
iii. OBLIQUE. From the iliopectineal eminence to the opposite sacro-iliac joint.
iv. SACROCOTYLOID. From the promontory of the sacrum to the iliopectineal eminence of

either side. It measures 9·5 cm (*see* Face
Presentation—Origin, p. 254).
v. DIAGONAL CONJUGATE DIAMETER.
Measured on vaginal examination from the
bottom of the symphysis pubis to the
promontory of the sacrum. It measures
12·5 cm. Subtraction of 1·5 cm gives an
approximation to the *true conjugate.*

b. *Mid-plane, or Plane of the Cavity, or Plane of Greatest Dimensions.* From the
middle of the back of the symphysis pubis to
the junction of the 2nd or 3rd pieces of the
sacrum.

c. *Plane of Least Dimensions*
DIAMETERS
i. ANTEROPOSTERIOR. From the lower border
of the back of the symphysis pubis to the
sacrococcygeal joint. The coccyx can be
ignored as it either bends or cracks out of the
way in labour.
ii. TRANSVERSE. Across the tips of the two
ischial spines—the *interischial spinous
diameter.*
Importance:
It is the level at which the axis of the pelvis
turns forwards. A hold-up at this level may
occasionally occur and require instrumental
assistance.

d. *Pelvic Outlet*
i. ANATOMICAL OUTLET
This is irregular in outline, consisting of two
triangles at an angle with each other but joined
across the ischial tuberosities.
TRACED FROM BEFORE BACKWARDS:
Under surface of the symphysis.
Inferior border of the ischiopubic rami.
Ischial tuberosities.
Sacrotuberous ligaments.
Tip of the coccyx.
N.B.   As these points are at different levels,
they do not represent an obstetrical plane.
ii. OBSTETRICAL OUTLET (more practical than
the anatomical concept).

TRACED FROM BEFORE BACKWARDS:
The point of contact anteriorly between the head and the pubic arch.
The inner aspect of the ischial tuberosities.
The sacrococcygeal joint.

DIAMETERS
i. ANTEROPOSTERIOR. *Posterior sagittal diameter* from the middle of the intertuberous diameter to the sacrococcygeal joint.
N.B.   This is not strictly correct but it is the nearest diameter with fixed endpoints for measuring.
ii. TRANSVERSE. *The intertuberous diameter.*

3. *Table of Pelvic Diameters*

	Antero-posterior	Oblique	Transverse
Brim	11 cm	12 cm	13·5 cm
Cavity	12 cm		12 cm
Plane of least dimensions	13·5 cm		11 cm
Outlet	8 cm		11 cm

4. *Walls of the Pelvis*
a. Anterior (4·5 cm): The pubic symphysis and rami.
b. Lateral: The iliac and ichial bones between the iliopectineal line and the tuberosity of the ischium.
c. Posterior (12 cm): The sacrum.
5. *Gaps in the Pelvis*
a. Obturator foramen.
b. Greater sacrosciatic foramen. Created from the notch by the sacrospinous ligament.
c. Lesser sacrosciatic foramen. Created from the notch by the sacrotuberous ligament.
6. *Ligaments*
a. Sacrospinous ligament—from the ischial spine to the lower margin of sacrum and coccyx.
b. Sacrotuberous ligament—from the ischial tuberosity to the lower margin of sacrum and coccyx.

7. *Pelvic Axis*

A curve, concave forwards, which angles fairly sharply at the plane of least dimensions.

8. *Pelvic Joints*

a. *Sacro-iliac joints* ⎫ Very little
b. *Symphysis pubis*   ⎬ movement.
c. *Sacrococcygeal joint* ⎭ May move quite freely.

9. *Variations in Pelvic Shape*

a. *Influences:*

Developmental—heredity (*see b. below*)

Acquired

   Mechanical, e.g. limps, scoliosis, lordosis, fracture.

   Disease, e.g. rickets, osteomalacia, tumours.

b. *Basic Hereditary Shapes of the Brim:*

Gynaecoid—rounded brim and a good pubic arch.

Anthropoid—anteroposterior diameter is larger than the transverse.

Android—shield-shaped pelvis with beaked forepelvis. The transverse diameter tends to be too far back to be fully utilized.

Platypelloid—or flat pelvis in which the anteroposterior diameter is reduced.

All these shapes may occur in large, average, or small sizes. The smaller sizes tend to 'funnel', i.e. the diameter gets proportionately less as the outlet is approached.

Soft Passages

1. *The Birth Canal*

a. Components: (1) Lower uterine segment (isthmus and cervix); (2) Vagina and vulva.

b. At full dilatation these form a single wide birth canal, curved forward along the pelvic axis and only narrowing at the vulva. It measures: anterior wall, 10 cm; posterior wall, 25 cm.

2. *Surrounding Structures*

a. *The pelvic floor muscles* are stretched to

form a gutter, which is of importance in causing internal rotation (q.v.).
b. The remaining pelvic organs are pulled out of the way by the *folding-door mechanism:*
The *bladder and urethra* are pulled upwards.
The *rectum and anus* are pushed downwards.
3. *Injury During Childbirth*
a. Laceration of the cervix.
b. Tearing apart of the muscles of the pelvic floor.
c. Laceration of the perineum.

Passengers

Fetus
1. *Weight*—average 3 kg at term. Tends to increase with parity.
2. *Disposition in Utero*
a. Attitude. The relationship of the fetal parts to one another (general flexion).
b. Lie. The relationship of the long axis of the fetus to that of the mother (longitudinal).
c. Presenting part. That part of the fetus reached by the finger during a vaginal examination (usually the vertex).
d. Level of the presenting part. Descriptive terms used:
High
At the brim ⎫ As the presenting
Engaged   ⎬ part descends.
Deeply engaged ⎭
N.B. The important question to answer is, 'Is the presenting part engaged or not?'
The mobility of the presenting part is only a factor which may assist in detecting the level. Note that if the pelvis is large the head may have some mobility even when fully engaged. Conversely, if the soft tissues are tense, there may be no mobility even when the presenting part is high. The term 'fixed' is ambiguous and is best avoided.
e. Position of the presenting part. The direction, around a vertical axis, in which the *denominator* points, e.g. left occipito-anterior.

The six positions of the vertex are:

1st position LOA ⎫
2nd position ROA ⎪ 'Classic' positions.
3rd position ROP ⎬
4th position LOP ⎭

LOL ⎫ Most frequent
ROL ⎬ positions, occurring
     ⎭ in 60% of cases.

N.B.   LOL = Left occipitolateral.

3. *Fetal Skull*

a. *Cranium and Base*

b. *Bones of the Cranium* (all formed from membrane)

Frontal bones (2).
Parietal bones (2).
Temporal bones (squamous portions) (2).
Occipital bone (squamous portion) (1).

c. *Sutures*

Frontal—between frontal bones.
Coronal—between frontal and parietal bones.
Sagittal—between parietal bones.
Lambdoidal—between parietal bones and the occiput.
Temporal—between parietal and temporal bones.

d. *Fontanelles*

ANTERIOR FONTANELLE OR BREGMA
Four sutures run into it: frontal, coronals (2), sagittal.

POSTERIOR FONTANELLE
Three sutures run into it: sagittal, lambdoidals (2).

SAGITTAL FONTANELLE
An uncommon dilatation of the sagittal suture which if not appreciated might lead to the mistaken diagnosis of: (1) Anterior fontanelle presentation (it lies too near the posterior fontanelle); or (2) Hydrocephalus (other sutures are normal).

e. *Regions*

VERTEX—between the anterior and posterior fontanelles.
SINCIPUT—in front of the bregma; may be

subdivided into: (1) *Brow*—between bregma
and nasion; or (2) *Face*—below the nasion.
OCCIPUT—behind the posterior fontanelle.

f. *Effect of Labour on Fetal Skull*

MOULDING = overlap and bending.
N.B. (*a*) The frontal bones and the occipital
bone slide under the parietals; (*b*) The anterior
parietal overrides the posterior.

CAPUT SUCCEDANEUM forms—oedema and
congestion in the area overlying the cervical
os. In vertex presentations the caput lies over
the anterior parietal bone, i.e. with the occiput
to the mother's left, over the right parietal
bone, and vice versa.

N.B. Cephalhaematoma is a swelling on the
baby's head produced by birth trauma. It
consists of haematoma lying between the
periosteum and the skull bone.

As the periosteum is adherent to the bone at
the suture lines, cephalhaematoma is limited
by the sutures, unlike caput succedaneum
which is not so restricted.

g. *Diameters* (*Fig.* 14)

SAGITTAL DIAMETERS IN VARIOUS
PRESENTATIONS:
Suboccipitobregmatic (9·5 cm), fully flexed
vertex presentation.
Suboccipitofrontal (10 cm), slightly deflexed
vertex association with posterior position
which undergoes the long internal rotation.
Occipitofrontal (11·5 cm), very deflexed   .
vertex associated with posterior position which
undergoes the short internal rotation.
Submentobregmatic (9·5 cm), fully extended
face presentation.
Submentovertical (11·5 cm), slightly
de-extended face presentation.
Mentovertical (13·5 cm), brow presentation.

CORONAL DIAMETERS IN VARIOUS
PRESENTATIONS:
Biparietal (9·5 cm): Passes the brim in a
lateral position of the vertex.

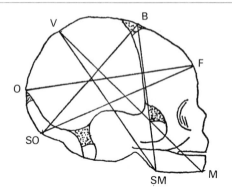

Fig. 14. Diameters of the fetal skull.

SO—B   Suboccipitobregmatic ⎫ Vertex
SO—F   Suboccipitofrontal   ⎬ diameters
O—F   Occipitofrontal   ⎭

SM—B   Submentobregmatic   ⎫ Face
SM—V   Submentovertical   ⎬ diameters

M—V   Mentovertical   Brow diameter

Bitemporal (8 cm): Passes the brim in a flat pelvis with a wide transverse.
Sub-supraparietal (8 cm): Passes the brim in asynclitism.

DIAMETERS DISTENDING THE VULVA AT FULL CROWNING:

1. Occipito-anterior delivery:
Suboccipitofrontal (10 cm)
Bitemporal (8 cm)

2. Occipitoposterior (face-to-pubes) delivery:
Occipitofrontal (11·5 cm)
Biparietal (9·5 cm).

3. Face delivery:
Submentovertical (11·5 cm)
Biparietal (9·5 cm).

N.B. The last two distend the vulva more than the occipito-anterior delivery and so need an episiotomy as a rule or a large tear will result.

4. *Fetal Trunk*
Bisacromial—12 cm (compressible).
Bitrochanteric—10 cm.
N.B.   Once the head has passed, the trunk
seldom gives difficulty. Occasionally large
shoulders can give dystocia.

The Remaining Passengers
1. Placenta.
2. Umbilical cord.
3. Liquor amnii.

17 Mechanism of Labour

EXPULSION OF THE FETUS IN ANTERIOR POSITIONS OF THE OCCIPUT (USING ONLY THE 'CLASSIC' POSITIONS)

All mechanisms can be given, with suitable modification, by the following basic formula—*which must be learnt:*

Descent
Flexion
Internal rotation
Extension
Restitution
External rotation
Lateral flexion of the trunk

Descent

Caused by the *powers* (q.v.).

Flexion

A general attitude; almost all joints are flexed.
1. Flexor muscle tone exceeds extensor muscle.
2. The effect of *uterine pressure* on the long axis of the fetus is to exaggerate the basic flexor attitude.

170

Internal Rotation

Rotation of the head inside the pelvis whereby the long axis of the fetal skull, the sagittal axis, is moved from the long oblique diameter of the brim by which it enters the pelvis to the long anteroposterior diameter of the outlet by which it leaves.

Caused by the *'gutter' action of the levator ani muscle.* The general rule is that *whichever part of the fetal head comes first into contact with the pelvic floor muscle, that part will be rotated forwards under the pubic arch.*

In the case of the anterior position of the occiput this part is the occiput which therefore rotates forwards one-eighth *of a circle or* 45°.

Extension

Extension of the head. As soon as the occiput is free of any resistance, having escaped from under the pubic arch, the *maternal soft parts pressing on the sinciput* cause the head to be thrown back and be delivered, the bregma, brow, face and chin sweeping over the perineum in turn.

Restitution

The shoulders are entering the brim in an oblique diameter (the opposite one to that occupied by the sagittal axis of the head). Internal rotation has placed a 45° twist on the neck. When the head has become free after extension *this twist is automatically undone.* Thus this process of restitution is in the opposite direction to that of internal rotation and of the same extent, i.e. 45° or one-eighth of a circle.

External Rotation

The movement made by the head outside the body, while the shoulders do an internal rotation of their own. It is also caused by the *'gutter' mechanism* and is through one-eighth of a circle, continuing the movement begun by restitution.

Lateral Flexion of the Trunk

The movement made as the child's body bends sideways round the *curved pelvic axis* and is swept round the pubis on to the mother's abdomen.

MECHANISM IN LATERAL POSITIONS OF THE OCCIPUT

Although William Smellie knew of the lateral positions, as is clear from his writings, he described no mechanism for these and neither has anyone since as far as the author knows. This is a surprising gap in our knowledge for in 60% of vertex presentations the head enters the brim in a lateral position.

Clearly, *internal rotations of the occiput* will be through 90° but what will the shoulder do? It seems unlikely that they will enter the brim in the anteroposterior diameter but will be deflected to one side or the other. The student can work out for him or herself how the mechanism will proceed with restitution and external rotation according to which side the posterior shoulder is deflected by the promontory. It will, of course, only be a theoretical exercise for there is probably no present evidence to support any conclusions.

MECHANISM OF THE THIRD STAGE

Separation of the Placenta

Caused by:
1. Reduction in size of the placental site which the less elastic placenta cannot follow so easily.
2. Retroplacental blood clot.

Expulsion of the Placenta

Two possible mechanisms—either may occur.
1. *Schultz's Method.* Applicable to fundal insertion. The placenta turns itself inside out,

assisted by retroplacental clot, and presents symmetrically at the vulva by its fetal surface.

2. *Matthews Duncan's Method.* Applicable to insertion on the lateral walls. The placenta slides out with one edge leading.

SOME INDICATIONS FOR CONFINEMENT IN A CONSULTANT UNIT

In general, every case except the perfectly normal one should be confined in a consultant unit, but the following instances may be specially mentioned:

Previous Obstetrical History

1. Primigravidae.
2. Four babies or more.
3. Postpartum haemorrhage or retained placenta.
4. Unexplained stillbirth.
5. Third degree tear or colporrhaphy.
6. Caesarean section or myomectomy.
7. Previous pre-eclampsia as a multigravida.
N.B. A previous simple outlet forceps delivery in a primigravida is not necessarily an indication for confinement in a consultant unit nor is mild or moderate pre-eclampsia as a primigravida when the blood pressure is normal early in a subsequent pregnancy.

Examination Findings

Associated Disease
1. Tuberculosis of lung or elsewhere.
2. Cardiac conditions.

3. Blood pressure over 130/80.
4. Diabetes mellitus.

Obstetrical Considerations
1. All women over 35.
2. The presence of Rh or other antibodies.
3. Contracted pelvis.

Conditions arising during Pregnancy

1. Failure of the head to engage at 36 weeks in a primigravida.
2. Breech presentation—in primigravida or multigravida.
3. Polyhydramnios.
4. Antepartum haemorrhage.
5. An unstable lie persisting to 38 weeks' gestation.
6. Postmaturity of 2 weeks.
7. Pre-eclampsia—however slight.
8. Multiple pregnancy.
9. Development of antibodies.

PREPARATIONS FOR ATTENDING A HOME CONFINEMENT

Preliminary Arrangements

The patient must be visited in her own home well beforehand to plan which room is to be used and to arrange water supply, heating, etc.

Equipment to be carried by the Midwife

This is not an exhaustive list. A few special points are mentioned for emphasis.

Drugs. (All these have been approved by the Central Midwives Board for use by midwives.)
1. *Analgesics*
a. Inhalation drugs.
 i. Nitrous oxide and oxygen (Entonox apparatus).
ii. Methoxyflurane (Penthrane) (Cardiff apparatus).
b. Oral preparations.
 i. Dichloralphenazone (Welldorm) 650 mg tablets.

ii. Pentazocine hydrochloride (Fortral) 50 mg capsules.

c. I.m. preparations.
  i. Pethidine 50 mg and 100 mg ampoules.
  ii. Pentazocine 30 mg ampoules.
  iii. Promazine hydrochloride (Sparine) 50 mg ampoules.

d. For infiltration. Lignocaine (without adrenaline) 0·5% 10 ml ampoules.

N.B.   All the above analgesics may be used by a midwife on her own initiative subject to approval by the Local Authority.

2. *Oxytocics*
a. Ergometrine tartrate in 0·5 mg ampoules.
b. Ergometrine maleate (0·5 mg) and oxytocin (5 units) in a combined ampoule (Syntometrine).

3. *For Neonatal Resuscitations*
Naloxone (Narcon Neonatal) 20 μg, ampoules of 1 ml.

4. *Antiseptics*
a. Chlorhexidine in cetrimide (Savlon) for skin sterilization and lotions.
b. Chlorhexidine (Hibitane) obstetric cream.

Other Equipment

1. *Sterile gowns, linen, and gloves* in pockets should be supplied by the local authority.
2. A *sphygmomanometer* should be in the equipment of *every* midwife.
3. A good quality *razor and blades* should be carried.

ONSET OF LABOUR

Symptoms

1. *Regular Contractions felt by the Patient*
N.B.   'False labour' may precede true labour by hours, or exceptionally days. It may be painful and differ only in that the contractions are not purposive so that dilatation of the cervix is not occurring. It differs from incoordinate labour (q.v.) only in that no cervical dilatation at all has occurred, so its

management is different (*see below*).

2. *A 'Show'* is a loss of a small quantity of bloodstained mucus. If it is more than this it must be regarded as antepartum haemorrhage and treated as such in particular, no vaginal examination may be done—just call medical aid.

3. *Loss of Liquor* may not mean the onset of labour, if there are no contractions, but the patient should send for the midwife or come into hospital.

Signs

1. *Regular Contractions observed by the Midwife.*
2. *Dilatation of the Cervix.*
3. *Bulging of the Membranes.*

EXAMINATION OF THE PATIENT DURING LABOUR

All results should be entered on a single chronological chart called a 'partograph' and nearly all are recorded graphically.

Observations to be recorded

The frequency of observations recommended is arbitrary and may be open to variation according to local views or the needs of the individual case or circumstances.

Maternal Condition
1. Maternal pulse—hourly in 1st stage; quarter-hourly in 2nd stage.
2. Blood pressure—hourly; more frequently if it is raised, perhaps even quarter-hourly.
3. Temperature—every 4 hours.
4. Urine—whenever passed or catheterized.

Fetal Condition
1. Fetal heart rate—quarter-hourly if not on monitor (*see* p. 187).
2. Liquor—record any change.
3. Moulding.

Progress of Labour
1. Dilatation of cervix in centimetres.
Examine vaginally every 3 hours at least.
2. Descent of the presenting part.
Record whenever a vaginal examination is performed.
3. Frequency of contractions—hourly at least.
4. Time when membranes rupture.

Oxytocic Drip (where applicable)—quarter-hourly. Record as mU/min or drops/min.

Analgesic Drugs (including epidural).

Object of these Observations

1. To detect failure of labour to progress steadily once it has become established and the cervix has begun to dilate. Once it has done so it is the dilatation of the cervix, as estimated on vaginal examination, that is the only reliable index of the progress of labour.

When it is clear that steady progress is not being made, an oxytocic drip is set up, but special care must be used in cases where there is danger of uterine rupture, e.g.:
a. 'Grand multipara'.
b. Previous Caesarean section.
c. Previous myomectomy.
2. To detect fetal distress in time to hasten delivery by forceps or Caesarean section.
3. To detect maternal distress.
a. A dextrose drip and sedatives may be required.
b. Unless normal delivery is not too far off, expedited delivery may be required.
c. Intrapartum eclampsia must be anticipated and prevented.

Vaginal Examination

When Necessary
1. On admission, or when first seen in labour.
2. Before giving sedation.
3. When the membranes rupture—especially if the presenting part is high when the examination should be done urgently.
4. When full dilatation is suspected.
5. If a cord complication is suspected, e.g. marked slowing of fetal heart during a contraction.
6. As a routine to record the progress of labour (*see above*).

Technique
1. For routine assessment of dilatation:
a. A sterile disposable glove should be put on by a 'no touch' technique.
b. After separating the labia, the skin should be wiped with cotton wool soaked in a solution of chlorhexidine 0·1% in cetrimide 1%.
c. Chlorhexidine obstetric cream should be used as a lubricant.
2. For an extensive vaginal examination: full aseptic ritual should be employed.

Findings
1. Vulva and vagina—discharge, moisture.
2. Cervix
a. Take-up and dilatation.
b. Thickness and oedema.
c. Softness.
d. Application to presenting part.
3. Membranes—intact or not; condition of liquor amnii.
4. Presenting part;
a. Identity (e.g. vertex, face, brow, breech, shoulder). The *vertex* is easily identified by its smooth outline, but diagnosis of the irregular presenting parts needs careful thought, and for each there is a characteristic feature for which the examiner must feel deliberately:
Face presentation—the gums.
Brow presentation—the orbital ridges.

Breech presentation—the anus.
Shoulder presentation—the ribs.
b. Caput formation and moulding.
c. Position (e.g. LOA, RSA, etc.)
d. Level or station (e.g. above or below the ischial spines, etc.).
e. Head fitting.
f. Descent during a contraction.
5. Pelvis
a. Diagonal conjugate (if presenting part is high enough).
b. Curve of the sacrum.
c. Prominence of the ischial spines.
6. Other findings
a. Cord (presentation or prolapse).
b. Placenta or vasa praevia.
c. Vaginal septum.
N.B.   Not all these possible findings should be sought in a routine examination purely to assess dilatation.

RELIEF OF PAIN

Properties of the Ideal Analgesic

1. Safe for mother and baby.
2. Gives effective relief of pain.
3. Must not interfere with the labour, i.e.:
a. No effect on uterine contractions.
b. Must not reduce the mother's ability to co-operate, i.e. she must not lose consciousness or control over herself.
N.B.   The ideal drug has not yet been discovered.

By Mouth

Dichloralphenazone (Welldorm) 650 mg tablets.
Dosage: 2–4 tablets.
Provides mild sedation and pain relief in early labour.

Pentazocine Hydrochloride (Fortral) 50 mg caps.
Dosage: 2 capsules.
More powerful effect in pain relief than dichloralphenazone.

Barbiturates

Among those most commonly used are:

1. *Amylobarbitone sodium* (Sodium Amytal) 200 mg (or up to 400 mg in special cases).

2. *Pentobarbitone sodium* (Nembutal) 200 mg

1. *Properties*

a. Not pain relievers.

b. May produce asphyxia neonatorum if given too near delivery.

2. *Uses*

a. To induce natural-like sleep, e.g. in antenatal cases or after delivery.

b. In conjunction with a pain reliever (such as morphine) to give a prolonged rest in labour, especially in inefficient uterine action.

c. To control the blood pressure in pre-eclamptics, antenatally and in labour, (sodium amytal is best for this).

By Intramuscular Injection

Morphine

1. *Properties*

a. It is the best pain-relieving drug we know and lasts for about 4 hours.

b. It does not necessarily induce sleep.

c. When the baby is born within 4 hours of morphine having been given it is liable to have its respiratory centre affected by the drug.

N.B. So long as the baby is in utero the drug is no danger to the fetus.

2. *Uses*

a. In primigravidae in the first stage. It is wise to do a vaginal examination before giving it, to avoid being misled about the degree of advancement of labour.

b. In cases of prolonged labour.

3. *Methods of Employment*

a. Alone.

b. In combination with:

i. Hyoscine (or scopolamine) 0·4 mg. Hyoscine has no analgesic effect itself but it potentiates that of morphine. If hyoscine be repeated, it prolongs the effect of the original

morphine: this was the basis of 'twilight sleep'.
ii. Nembutal 200 mg (or other barbiturates).
Gives sleep as well as relief from pain, e.g. in
prolonged labour.

Pethidine
1. *Dosage.* 150 mg is the usual dose but up to
200 mg can be given. The total amount a
midwife can give on her own in any one
labour and the amount of the drug she can
hold is determined by the individual Local
Authority.
50 mg can be given by intravenous injection
for quick action, but it should be given slowly
as it often produces vomiting if given quickly.
2. *Properties*
a. Less effective than morphine and lasts for
about 2 hours.
b. It is safer for the baby, if full term, even if
given near delivery.
3. *Uses*
a. In multigravidae when in good first-stage
labour.
b. In primigravidae when it is too late for
morphine to be given with safety.
4. *Methods of Employment*
a. Alone.
b. In combination with:
 i. Hyoscine—as above for morphine.
 ii. Promazine hydrochloride (Sparine)—
25 mg potentiates the pethidine and relieves
anxiety and nausea.
iii. Promethazine hydrochloride (Phenergan)—
25 mg i.m., potentiates the pethidine.

Pentazocine Hydrochloride (Fortral)
1. *Dosage* 30–45 mg
2. *Properties:*
a. Similar to pethidine in effectiveness.
b. Similar to pethidine in its effect on the
baby.
c. Addiction is rare.
d. Should not be given to patients on
monoamine-oxidase inhibitors.

e. May produce dizziness and mental disturbance.

By Inhalation

Advantages. Quick action and quick disappearance of effects.

Disadvantage. Patients vary in their response so that a fixed concentration that is never likely to produce unconsciousness in any patient will be ineffective on some patients. This is the dilemma of those who design apparatus for midwives to use, and they have not solved the problem completely.

Drugs
1. Nitrous oxide and oxygen mixture (50% N_2O and 50% oxygen mixed in one cylinder). The Entonox apparatus has been approved.
2. Methoxyflurane (Penthrane)—administered by the Cardiff inhaler which has been approved by the Central Midwives Board. (Now seldom used.)

Block Analgesia

1. *Local Infiltration.* Using lignocaine (Xylocaine) 0·5%.
2. *Pudendal Block.* Using lignocaine 0·5%.
3. *Epidural*
Advantage: Complete relief of pain without adverse effect on uterine action or fetus.
Disadvantages:
a. Requires the attendance of a highly trained anaesthetist to insert the catheter.
b. Failures occur—about 80% of cases get satisfactory analgesia.
c. The procedure may have to be abandoned, e.g. dural tap or bloody tap. The former may give rise to severe headache and requires 48 hours lying flat on the back.
d. Complications may occur—mostly minor (e.g. headache, backache and soreness at needle site, bladder disturbance) but rarely serious (e.g. paraplegia).

e. Instrumental delivery rate is doubled.

Conclusion:

The technique is very useful where patients are suffering pain which is inadequately controlled by other means. It is unjustified for routine use unless there are sufficient senior anaesthetists able to devote an appreciable amount of their time to performing and supervising epidural techniques. Only thus can the success rate be maintained and the incidence of complications kept sufficiently low.

Antidote to Morphine, Pethidine and Pentazocine

Naloxone Hydrochloride (Narcan)

1. *Use.* When morphine has been given within 4 hours of the imminent birth of the baby or pethidine has been given within 1 hour. It prevents or treats neonatal asphyxia caused by the respiratory depression produced by these drugs.

2. *Methods of Employment*

a. To the mother—0·4 mg in 1 ml intramuscularly. Has to be within 20 min of the birth of the baby to be effective.

b. To the baby—*Narcan Neonatal*, 30 μg in 1·5 ml (or 10 μg/kg) into the cord, intramuscularly or subcutaneously.

3. *Additional Points*

a. Nalaxone is *not* an antidote to barbiturates.

b. Pethidine is sometimes given simultaneously with an antidote (in this case *levallorphan*—the combined ampoule is *Pethilorfan*). This would seem to be illogical and unnecessary, for:

a. Pethidine is not very depressing to the respiration.

b. The antidote may reduce the analgesic effect too.

c. The antidote can be given in those cases where the need arises.

Regulations Affecting Midwives in the Use of Drugs

The Central Midwives Board Regulations state that a midwife must only administer drugs, including analgesics, in the use of which she has been thoroughly instructed in the course of her training, whether before or after enrolment, and with whose dosage and methods of administration or application she is familiar.

Community Midwife (*see* pp. 175, 176)

Hospital Midwife
Unlike the Community Midwife, the Hospital Midwife must follow the normal hospital practice of having all drugs she gives signed for by a doctor. However, in order to avoid undue delay in treating the patient the authorized procedure is for a list of drugs, which the midwife can give on her own authority, to be agreed between the medical and midwifery staff. This list is to be displayed in the labour ward. Nevertheless for any drug administered a counter-signature from a doctor must be obtained within 12 hours.

Such a list might be as follows, this one being that in use at St James's University Hospital, Leeds, but each hospital will have its own list:
1. *Analgesics*
Pethidine 100 mg i.m. up to 200 mg.
Promethazine Hydrochloride (Phenergan) 25 mg i.m.
Promazine Hydrochloride (Sparine) 50 mg i.m.
Welldorm 650–1950 mg orally.
2. *For Episiotomy*
Lignocaine (without adrenaline) 1% up to 10 ml.
3. *Analgesia on Lying-in Ward*
Paracetamol 0·5–1 g orally.
4. *Third Stage*
Syntometrine 1 ml i.m.
Ergometrine 0·5 mg i.m. (0·25 mg i.v. in an emergency).

The Grantly Dick-Read Theory and Psychoprophylaxis

Although opinion is divided as to the actual relief of pain obtained, it is generally accepted that physical and mental relaxation, achieved by gaining the patient's confidence and abolishing fear by means of reasoned explanation, goes far towards making what pain there is less of a trial.

Nevertheless, the concept of Natural Childbirth in which the patient is encouraged to do without analgesia should not be carried too far. If or when the degree of pain is becoming unacceptable the labouring woman should be encouraged to accept some method of pain relief; it can be regarded as a supplement to her relaxation techniques not as a replacement for them.

MANAGEMENT IN LABOUR

First Stage

Bowels. A saline enema should be given early in labour.

Posture during Labour. During the first stage the mother should walk about and carry on with duties which will distract her attention for as long as possible. This can be alternated with sitting and short periods lying down. *This applies in hospital as well as at home,* however much more simple it is administratively for all patients to be kept in bed.

Duration. Do not prophesy to the patient or her relatives how long labour will take.

Nutrition. Give nothing by mouth once labour is established other than mouthwashes and small sips of fluid. Solid food may be dangerous if an anaesthetic has to be given (inhalation vomit is an important cause of maternal death and food stays a long time in the stomach of the pregnant woman): only a large stomach tube can remove solid food before an anaesthetic.

The Bladder must be kept empty.

Medical Aid must be sought by the midwife for all abnormalities.
1. Failure of labour to progress.
2. Any antepartum haemorrhage.
3. Presentation or prolapse of the cord.
4. Abnormal presentation, e.g. breech.
5. Fetal distress:
a. Meconium-stained liquor.
b. Fetal heart rate: (1) Steadily rising or exceeding 160, (2) A fall of 20 beats/min or below 120.

Fetal Monitoring
1. *Use.* On all high-risk cases if available and on other cases as the obstetrician indicates.

Some think it may be useful for all cases, but there may be doubt whether this would improve results. In any case it is advisable for a labouring woman not to be immobilized by drips and monitors without good reason; it is better that she should be able to walk about.
2. *Methods*
a. Fetal electrocardiography
b. Ultrasonic Doppler cardiography
These are recorded on a cardiotocograph i.e. recording both fetal heart rate and uterine contractions.
3. *Types of Abnormality*
a. Rate *rises above 160 beats*/min or *falls below 120.* A steady rise or fall even before these limits is a warning.
b. *Type I dip.* Rate falls below 120 at the onset of a contraction but returns quickly to normal at its end—probably normal, but watch.
Type II dip. Rate falls below 120 beginning well after the onset of the contraction and returning only slowly to normal well after its end—serious fetal distress.
c. *Loss of beat-to-beat variation,* i.e. a very flat trace—a warning, but combined with other signs is significant.

Fetal Scalp Blood Sampling
1. *Use.* To try and exclude fetal hypoxia and save an unnecessary Caesarean section when this method of delivery is being contemplated as a result of equivocal fetal heart monitoring.
2. *Method.* Blood is taken from the fetal scalp via a special conical speculum and its pH is measured.
3. *Results.* pH greater than 7·25—baby is satisfactory; less than 7·2—fetal distress; 6·9 or less—fetal death is imminent.

Second Stage

Clinical Evidence that the Second Stage has begun
1. Contractions become stronger and more frequent.
2. Patient gets an involuntary urge to bear down, associated with a grunting respiration caused by closure of the glottis.
3. Bulging of the perineum with each contraction.
4. On vaginal examination the cervix is fully dilated.

Conduct of the Second Stage
1. The patient *must never be left alone* during the second stage or even the end of the first.
2. Fetal heart rate is taken every quarter hour or even after each contraction.
3. Delay encouraging the patient to bear down until the head is visible and is quite low: it is better to start her pushing late rather than early.
4. Keep the bladder empty.

Conduct of Delivery
1. *Controlling the Head. Objects:*
a. To prevent severe laceration which rapid delivery during a contraction would cause.

b. To prevent the head extending until the occiput is free, i.e. so that it is only the suboccipito-frontal diameter which distends the vulva.

2. *Positions for Delivery* (both methods should be practised):

a. Left Lateral:

Good view of perineum.

Avoids the sagging centre of a poor bed.

b. Dorsal:

Easier for the patient to push.

No need to move her for the third stage.

3. *Shoulder Dystocia.* A baby can be lost if the shoulders fail to deliver within 7 to 10 minutes. The first indication of the shoulders not entering the brim is given by failure of the chin to escape over the perineum, which has to be 'milked' back.

Action to be taken by the midwife:

a. Send for medical aid.

b. Attempt to achieve delivery by: (1) Reasonable traction on the head, but beware Erb's palsy. (2) Fundal pressure. (3) Pressure on the anterior shoulder, above the pubis.

N.B. The position of the caput (q.v.) may indicate the way the head should restitute.

c. Prepare a trolley for the doctor

Third Stage

Management of the Newborn Baby

1. Place the baby with head well below the rest of the body.

2. Suck out mucus if possible *before* the first breath.

3. Tie the cord when pulsation has ceased (this is a controversial point and need not be pressed if other factors make it difficult to achieve).

A double ligature is used and repeated glances to detect bleeding, must be made.

4. Apgar score—to assess fetal asphyxia. Record at 1 minute, and 5 minutes.

Score	0	1	2
Heart rate	Absent	Below 100/min	Over 100/min
Respiratory effort	Absent	Weak cry Hypoventilation	Strong cry
Muscle tone	Limp	Some flexion of limbs	Active movement Limbs well flexed
Reflex response to nasal catheter	None	Grimace	Cry
Colour body limbs	Blue Pale	Pink Blue	Completely pink

0–2 points: severe depression
3–6 points: moderate depression
7–10 points: good condition

5. *Resuscitation*
At Birth if pulse is less than 100/min, intubate.
a. Use laryngoscope.
b. Aspirate larynx and trachea.
c. Pass tube 2 cm into trachea.
d. Give puffs of oxygen every 2 sec using a blow-off valve set at 20 cm of water.
At One Minute if spontaneous respirations not established—
　i. *Peripheral Stimulation.* If no success in 1 min:
　ii. *Airway, Bag and Mask:* Give puffs every 2 sec using a blow-off valve set at 20 cm of water (not very effective).
　iii. *Intubate* if spontaneous respirations are not established quickly.

When Apgar reaches 7–10 no further action.

Management of the Third Stage
1. Turn the mother on to her back, if she has been delivered in the left lateral position.
2. *Signs that the Placenta is in the Vagina*
a. A gush of blood accompanies separation of the placenta.
b. 'Lengthening' of the cord.
c. The uterus has: Risen higher and fallen to

one side; become harder and smaller (like a cricket ball).

d. Test for Expulsion. With one hand placed between the pubis and the fundus, push the latter upwards; meanwhile the other hand holds the cord on light tension. If the cord runs into the vagina the placenta is still within the uterus; if not it is in the vagina.

3. *Time taken by Various Oxytocics to Produce an Effect*

Ergometrine intramuscularly	7 min
Ergometrine and Hyalase intramuscularly	4¾ min

(These are supplied as two separate ampoules which are mixed in the syringe prior to injection.)

Oxytocin intramuscularly	2½ min
Ergometrine intravenously	41 sec

4. *Conservative Management of the Third Stage*

a. One hand is placed on the fundus, exerting only gentle pressure and moving only enough to detect changes in uterine height and shape. *Objects:*

To *detect and control haemorrhage*—prevents clot collection in the vagina by preventing the fundus rising. To *detect the spontaneous separation* of the placenta and its *expulsion into the vagina.*

b. Once lying in the vagina the placenta can be finally expelled:

By the *mother's secondary powers* (does not always succeed) or

By *using the contracted fundus as a plunger* the attendant can expel the placenta through the vulva.

The conservative management of the third stage is that which for generations had been taught to doctors and midwives in the belief that any more active procedure might lead to occasional incidents of acute puerperal inversion of the uterus, by pressure being exerted on the fundus, or by traction on the cord, when the uterus was flaccid.

5. *Active Management of the Third Stage* (controlled cord traction or Brandt-Andrews manoeuvre). (Brandt M. L. (1933) *Am. J. Obstet. Gynecol.,* **25,** 662; Andrews C. J. (1940) *South Med. & Surg.,* **102,** 605.)
a. An oxytocic is given when the head is crowned, when the anterior shoulder is born, or after complete delivery of the baby, but while the placenta is still in situ. The choice of timing and of the oxytocic preparation is still debated.
Ergometrine given intravenously with the delivery of the anterior shoulder of the baby has been established as being the most effective technique, but is difficult to achieve by a single-handed attendant.
A mixture of *ergometrine* 0·5 *mg and oxytocin* 5 *units (Syntometrine) given intramuscularly during, or immediately after, delivery of the baby* is the best compromise: the oxytocin gives a quick action and the ergometrine a prolonged one (first suggested by M. P. Embrey (1961) *Br. Med. J.* **1,** 1737).
b. With the ensuing contraction the cord is held with one hand and the uterus is pushed upwards per abdomen: the procedure is similar to that used as a 'Test for Expulsion' (*see above*), but the cord is not allowed to run into the vagina so that the placenta is pulled out of the uterus.
(In the original descriptions by Brandt the placenta is allowed to descend into the lower segment and vagina before interfering; but most people now do not wait for this, attempting to pull the placenta out of the uterus as soon as a good contraction has occurred.)
c. Once in the vagina the placenta is expelled by using the contracted uterus as a plunger, assisted by cord traction.
Advantages
The third stage is shortened.

The PPH rate may be reduced.
Danger. If traction is exerted with the uterus flaccid, acute puerperal inversion may occur, but if the uterus is contracted the cord will snap before this occurs, the only disadvantage being the mess and that there will no longer be anything to pull on!
The active management has virtually replaced the conservative one.

Duties after Delivery

Ergometrine
0·5 mg intramuscularly may be given if it has not been given already.

Examination of the Placenta
1. Missing succenturiate lobes—vessels on edge.
2. Gaps on the maternal surface or missing membrane: not very reliable.
3. Presence of haemorrhage, infarcts, etc.
4. Examine the cut cord for the number of arteries present. If only one, there is a high chance of an abnormality of the urinary tract.
N.B.   Record these in notes.

Send Cord Blood to the Laboratory if:
1. Mother is Rh negative.
2. Any antibodies are present in the maternal serum.
Tests performed are:
1. Coombs' test.
2. Haemoglobin estimation.
3. Serum bilirubin.
4. Blood grouping.

Lacerations
1. Degrees
First Degree—skin and vaginal epithelium only.
Second Degree—muscle of the pelvic floor is involved.
Third Degree—involves the anal sphincter at least and may spread up into anal canal and rectum.

Central perineal tear—the tear begins midway between fourchette and anus. (It must be completed towards the fourchette at once to save the anal sphincter.)

2. *Repair*

a. Small tears involving skin, vaginal epithelium and subcutaneous tissue only, up to a diameter of about 3 cm, are better not repaired: (1) There is less pain. (2) The healing is more natural and avoids the fold of skin in the perineum which so often causes dyspareunia. (3) A tear in the next labour will probably be avoided. A long experience following this policy of leaving the majority of first degree tears unsutured has confirmed the validity of this approach.

b. Good light is essential.

c. Local anaesthetic must be used.

A continuous catgut suture approximates the vaginal edges.

Interrupted catgut sutures unite the levatores ani and deep tissues of the perineum.

Non-absorbable sutures or a subcuticular stitch is used for the perineal skin.

Settling the Patient Down

1. Do not leave the patient until one hour after delivery.

2. Watch for haemorrhage concealed in the vagina.

3. Instruct the mother to keep her fist pressed on to the fundus.

Further Care of the Baby

1. Inspect for abnormalities, e.g.:

Hydrocephaly.

Cleft palate and hare lip.

Facial palsy.

Mongolism.

Meningocele, myelocele, etc.

Hernia—umbilical and inguinal.

Webbed fingers, extra digits, etc.

Erb's palsy.

Talipes, accessory toes, etc.

Urethra—e.g. hypospadias.
Undescended testes.
Any evidence of dubious sex.
Imperforate anus.
Test for congenital dislocation of the hip.
2. Oil and bath the baby at 40° C.
3. Apply a clip to the cord (if this has not been done already). Make sure it is not too close to the abdominal wall, for bleeding between the clip and abdominal wall is difficult to control.
4. On sixth day of life, perform on the baby:
a. Guthrie test for *phenylketonuria, and*
b. Test for *neonatal hypothyroidism.*
Method: Four drops of blood are dropped on to circles of absorbent paper on a special card.

BACTERIOLOGY

Bacteria can be considered as:
1. Pathogenic (harmful to man).
2. Non-pathogenic.
Distribution of bacteria is said to be ubiquitous. No surface or atmosphere, unless it be specially treated, is free from organisms. Fortunately they are mostly non-pathogenic.

Classification

By shape and staining. *Gram stain* consists in the application in sequence of:
Methyl violet.
Lugol's iodine (fixes the methyl violet).
Alcohol (removes methyl violet from Gram-negative bacteria).
Neutral red (stains red those organisms decolorized by alcohol).
Therefore: Gram-positive organisms remain blue.
Gram-negative organisms stain red.

	Shape and Grouping	Staining	Disease (Examples)
a. COCCI (DOTS)			
i. Staphylococci	Clusters of dots	Gram-positive	Boils and pimples

		Shape and Grouping	Staining	Disease (Examples)
ii.	Streptococci	Chains of dots	Gram-positive	Sore throat: cellulitis
iii.	Diplococci	Pairs of dots		
	(1) Gonococci		Gram-negative	Gonorrhoea: ophthalmia
	(2) Pneumo-cocci		Gram-positive	Pneumonia
	(3) Meningo-cocci		Gram-negative	Cerebrospinal meningitis
b.	BACILLI (RODS)			
i.	*E. coli*	Clusters of minute rods	Gram-negative	Pyelitis: pelvic abscess
ii.	Tubercle	Clusters of minute rods	Acid-fast	Pulmonary tuberculosis
iii.	*Cl. welchii*	Large rods	Gram-positive	Gas gangrene
c.	SPIROCHAETES			
		Spirals	Seen by dark ground illumination, unstained	Syphilis

TRANSMISSION OF DISEASE

Sources

Autogenous
1. Endogenous (from genital tract).
2. Exogenous (from elsewhere in the body).

Heterogenous
1. Other patients.
2. Attendants.
3. Visitors.
4. Husband.
5. Animals (e.g. tuberculosis from milk).

Vectors

1. Droplet.
2. Dust (includes some droplet infection).
3. Direct contact, e.g. hands, instruments, dressings, bedpans, bath, coitus, etc.
4. Water and food, e.g. dysentery.
5. Animals.

Portals

1. Lungs and pharynx, e.g. tuberculosis, pneumonia, tonsillitis.
2. Mouth, e.g. tuberculosis, dysentery.
3. Intact skin or mucous membrane, e.g. syphilis.
4. Wounds and raw areas:
a. Injury, e.g. perineal tears.
b. Surgical wounds, e.g. episiotomy, abdominal incisions.
c. Placental site.

LESIONS PRODUCED BY CERTAIN BACTERIA

	General Disease	*Pelvic Lesions*
1. Haemolytic streptococcus (droplet mainly)	*a.* Scarlet fever *b.* Tonsillitis *c.* Septicaemia *d.* Some connection with nephritis	Little to be seen. Serves as a portal of entry with little local damage
2. Anaerobic strepto-coccus (often endogenous)		*a.* Abscess and cellulitis *b.* Thrombophlebitis
3. Staphylococcus (direct contact; dust)	Pimples and boils	Localized suppura-tion
	(It is typical of the staphylococcus that it stimulates the body to wall off the lesion)	
4. *E. coli* (direct contact)	Cystitis and pyelitis	Collection of fetid pus
5. Gonococcus (direct contact)	Ophthalmia neonato-rum	Vaginitis; salpingitis (rare in pregnancy and puerperium)
6. *Cl. welchii* (direct contact; dust)	(Lives and grows deep in tissue devitalized by trauma where it can be cut off from the air, e.g. compound fractures of thigh, endometritis, metritis, and parametritis.)	

PROPHYLAXIS

Pregnancy

1. Improve general health, especially anaemia.
2. Treat and clear up all septic lesions.

3. Avoid contamination of the vagina in the *last month* of pregnancy by:
a. Advising against coitus.
b. Only performing a sterile vaginal examination.

Delivery

1. Avoid trauma.
2. Treat retained products of conception.
3. Careful observance of a sterile technique (*see below*).

Hospital Routine

Avoid Droplet Infection
1. Exclude streptococcal and staphylococcal carriers:
a. Healthy carriers detected by swabbing.
b. Cases of sore throat.
N.B. Visitors should be asked to stay away if they have a sore throat.
2. Exclude all attendants with septic skin lesions, etc.
3. Use masks whenever the vulva is exposed in the labour ward.
4. Restrict the number of visitors.

Avoid Dust Infection
1. *Blankets*
a. Never shake them on the ward; handle gently.
b. A ward blanket should never cross the threshold of the theatre or labour ward.
c. The handling of the blankets by the laundry should be such as to ensure sterilization. Cotton cellular blankets can be boiled without 'felting' as woollen ones do.
2. *Floors.* Only a wet-sweeping or vacuum technique should be employed. The use of antiseptic solutions, later removed by a wet-vacuum machine, may be helpful.
3. Masks should be worn if the vulva is exposed. Anything more than this, but short of a complete change with the donning of gowns, boots, etc., is a mere gesture to convention but will do nothing to reduce cross infection.

4. *Dirty Dressings* should never be done on a main ward: the patient should be moved to a side ward reserved for the purpose.

Avoid Spread by Hands and Instruments
1. *On the Ward*
'No touch' swabbing technique is taught to lying-in patients who are up. (1) Bed-pans are sterilized. (2) Toilet seats must be disinfected before and after use.
2. *Theatre and Labour Ward*
a. Normal scrubbing-up and gowning technique should apply, be it in labour ward or theatre, for delivery.
b. Care in movement, etc., in theatre. Movements should not be hurried. Even experienced people are guilty of breaches of theatre technique, such as touching the corners of the coverings of sterile trolleys with non-sterile clothing as they walk by.
c. Skin sterilization:
Patient under general anaesthetic—use 70% spirit with 0·5% chlorhexidine; it will be effective in under 1 min.
Conscious patients—use 1% cetrimide with 0·5% chlorhexidine, but sterilization is not perfect even after waiting for 5 minutes.

Isolation of Septic or Potentially Septic Cases as well as known healthy carriers.

20

Physiology of the Puerperium

DEFINITION

The *puerperium* is the period required for the organs to return to normal after delivery—about six weeks. The changes are most marked in the first two weeks of the *lying-in period.*

LOCAL CHANGES

Uterus

Involution of the Uterus

1. *Condition Immediately after Delivery*

a. Fundus 13 cm above the pubis (rises to 15 cm after a few hours).

b. Size:

Length—20 cm.

Cavity—15 cm long.

Walls—5 cm thick in the upper segment.
   1 cm thick in the lower segment.

c. Weight—1000 g.

2. *Changes.* Weight returns to between 50–70 g in six weeks by a process of *autolysis,* the surplus protein in the muscle fibres being broken down and excreted: no actual destruction of muscle cells occurs.

Fifty per cent of the weight loss is in the 1st week.

Twenty-five per cent of the weight loss is in the 2nd week.
Twenty-five per cent of the weight loss is in the remaining four weeks.

The Endometrium splits off through the spongy layer and is shed. A new endometrium is formed in the next three weeks, except at the placental site.

The Placental Site is a raised area of thrombosed sinuses and fibrin after birth. It is undermined by the developing endometrium and cast off, the area being finally covered by regenerated endometrium by the 7th week.

The Cervix
First few days—admits 2 fingers easily.
Seventh day—internal os closed.
Fourteenth day—external os closed, but remains permanently as a transverse slit.

Lochia

Constituents
1. Red and white corpuscles.
2. Degenerating epithelial cells and decidua.
3. Mucus.
4. Bacteria.

Changes
Lochia rubra, 0–5th day.
Lochia serosa, 6th–10th day.
Lochia alba, 11th–15th day.
This classic description is open to wide variation, red lochia often persisting until the 7th or 10th day, and coloured lochia until the 24th.

Vagina

Rugae reappear in 3rd week.

Other Structures

1. Peritoneum.
2. Abdominal wall.
3. Pelvic floor muscles.
4. Parametrium.

These all involute to near their original state, but some relaxation may persist, especially in the pelvic floor and parametrium.

GENERAL CHANGES

Blood

1. The *hydraemia* of pregnancy goes, the *red cell* count and *haemoglobin* content returning to normal.
2. The *leucocytosis* of labour goes.

Urine

A big increase in output occurs in the first few days of the puerperium.

Hormones

1. Oestrogen ⎫
2. Gonadotrophin ⎬ Fall to normal low level.
3. Progesterone secretion ceases.

LACTATION

Cause of Lactation

1. *Oestrogen and Progesterone* prepare the breasts during pregnancy.
2. *Prolactin* is released at birth by the pituitary, to start lactation.
3. *Sucking* by the baby is the stimulus which keeps lactation going and so long as the baby sucks no hormonal adminstration can stop lactation.

Colostrum

This only occurs in the first *two days*.

Content
1. Serum albumin.
2. Colostrum corpuscles (degenerating epithelial cells).
3. Salts.
4. Fat globules (less than in milk).

Milk

Milk occurs on the *3rd day*. Often associated with:
1. Local discomfort or pain.
2. Headaches.
3. A rise of temperature (occasionally quite a high one), which has settled to normal completely by the next day.

21

Management of the Puerperium

OBSERVATIONS

To detect the earliest signs of abnormality.

Temperature

May indicate sepsis, but note the frequent pyrexia at the onset of lactation which settles at once.

Pulse Rate

A rise, even a slight one, may be a better indication of trouble than the temperature chart. It may indicate:
1. Sepsis.
2. Anaemia—a persistently raised rate.
3. Thrombosis—a minor rise at about the 10th day.

Blood Pressure

Record fairly frequently for the first 6 days of the puerperium, especially in cases with known pre-eclampsia, with special attention to the 'rebound' phenomenon on or about the 4th day (*see* p. 100).

Height of the Fundus

This is of no practical help in assessing progress of involution, but it ensures a daily abdominal palpation, which will help to detect a distended bladder or gross constipation. It is said to be 15 cm above the pubis on the first day and falls on the average 1 cm daily, disappearing after a fortnight.

Lochia

Variations from the average are wide (*see* p. 202), but:

1. Continued bright red loss or recurrence once it has cleared up suggest retained products of conception and the neccessity for curettage.

N.B.   Significant amounts of placental material are not always found, however. An ultrasound examination may exclude the presence of retained products of conception and thereby save the patient an unnecessary exploration of the uterus.

2. Offensive lochia suggests intra-uterine sepsis.

Anaemia

Common after delivery. Perform haemoglobin estimations when in doubt.

Thrombosis in Legs

May occur from the 6th day onwards (most frequently about the 10th). Watch must be kept for *pain in the calf* or in the *thigh*, associated with *oedema*. It is important to detect this in its earliest stages and any *mild rise in temperature or pulse rate* warrants a search for thrombosis.

REST, EXERCISES AND AMBULATION

Rest

Rest in adequate amounts in the early days after delivery is necessary to recover from the effort of childbearing.

Sedation

Sedation is often necessary (e.g. Diazepam 2–5 mg or sodium amytal 200 mg), for tired though she may be, the excitement may prevent the patient sleeping.

Sleep
Eight hours at night plus a 'nap' in the afternoon. (Noisy babies should be kept in the nursery at night even though they spend much of the day alongside their mothers.)
N.B.   Inadequate rest may predispose to *puerperal insanity.*

Postnatal Exercises

Objects. To prevent:
1. Thrombosis and embolism by keeping the blood moving.
2. Loss of muscular tone.

Start after first 24 hours.

Rising

Unless there is some medical reason, e.g. heart disease, why the patient should be confined to bed, the delivered woman can be up and about at once and should be encouraged to do so.

Advantages
1. Reduction in thrombosis and embolism.
2. Maintains muscular tone.
3. Ensures a quicker return to full vigour both mentally and physically.

Disadvantages
1. Toilet, washing and showering or bathing facilities are often inadequate.
2. The danger of cross-infection from bath or toilet seats must be borne in mind. Antiseptics such as 'Savlon' should be used on the seats.

Technique
When the delivered woman is out of bed she should be walking most of the time. Sitting in a chair is the worst position for the postpartum or postoperative patient as it restricts the circulation in the legs and predisposes to thrombosis and embolism. 'Out of bed for bed-making' in the sense of sitting in a chair is a

step backwards rather than forwards. When not walking a patient should lie on top of or in bed where more generalized body support is afforted.

CARE OF NIPPLES

After each feed, dry the nipple, apply lanoline, protect with a small piece of lint, and support the breast with a loose binder.

DIET

As for pregnancy. Free drinking of fluids is often advocated to aid milk production, but is probably ineffective.

BLADDER

1. Reflex postpartum retention may occur, especially if there are lacerations. Therefore, careful watch should be kept on output in the first day or two and the abdomen palpated for an over-distended bladder.
2. If retention is occurring then proceed as follows:
a. Try persuasion.
b. Pour warm fluid over the vulva.
c. Turn on taps.
d. Allow her to get out of bed and use a bed-pan on a stool, or chair.
e. Carbachol i.m. may be ordered.
f. Catheterization is a last resort, but should not be delayed until overdistension has caused the bladder to lose its tone.
3. If persistent retention occurs, an 'indwelling catheter' may be inserted and drained into a bottle for 24 hours until the bladder regains its tone.

If an indwelling catheter is necessary it should be 'covered' by an appropriate antibiotic.

AFTER-PAINS

After-pains due to uterine contraction to expel clot, etc., may be painful enough to require sedatives, e.g. aspirin, paracetamol etc.

INVOLUTION OF THE UTERUS

1. *This is Delayed by:* (i) Sepsis; (ii) Retained placental fragments.
2. *Curettage* may be called for to deal with the bleeding caused by such fragments.
3. *Ergometrine* is probably valueless in influencing involution (Chassar Moir).
4. *Subinvolution* is the term used to describe a uterus which has remained bulky due to incomplete involution. The tendency is, however, to regard its clinical significance as being open to doubt.

MENTAL STATE—FOURTH DAY 'GLOOMS'

An intense state of depression, sudden in onset and in departure, lasting for about one day only—usually the fourth day—is so common that it is worth warning the delivered woman that it is likely to occur and disappear by the next day. More prolonged changes in mental state should be regarded as a warning of possible puerperal insanity.

DISCHARGE FROM HOSPITAL

In the absence of any medical indication for remaining in hospital, and providing home arrangements are suitable, discharge from hospital at about 48 hours after delivery is the most popular time. However, there is no theoretical objection to discharge within hours of delivery if arrangements can be made.

In all cases leaving hospital there must be good liaison between the hospital and the community midwife to ensure continuity of supervision.

22 Complications of the Puerperium

PUERPERAL PYREXIA

Not all puerperal sepsis will lead to a significant rise in temperature so that other clinical features, e.g. pulse rate, the general condition of the patient, etc., must be considered to be of equal if not greater importance.

Calling Medical Aid by the Midwife

Standards laid down by the Central Midwives Board:
That during the lying-in period after abortion or childbirth there should be:
1. A temperature of 37·4°C. on three successive days.
2. A temperature of 38°C. on one occasion.
3. A persistently raised pulse rate.
N.B. Under Semmelweiss in 1843 1 hospital case in 3 died, mainly from sepsis.

PUERPERAL SEPSIS

Genital

Source, Vector and Portal (*See* Chapter 19)

Factors Favouring Infection
1. *Resistance*
a. *General*
Haemorrhage.

Anaemia.
Malnutrition.
These do not cause infection but make it a more serious matter should it occur.
b. Local
Trauma.
Retained products of conception.
2. *Organisms*
a. Invasiveness and virulence.
b. Resistance to antibiotics.
Type of Lesion depends upon the organism. (*See* Chapter 19.)
Site of Lesion. Consider the anatomical structures in ascending order:

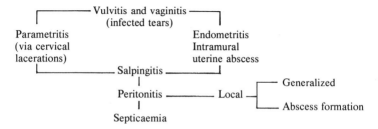

Clinically
1. General signs of infections (e.g. pyrexia, raised pulse rate, etc.)
2. Localizing signs (e.g. pain, offensive vaginal discharge, etc.).

Extra-genital   **Respiratory Tract,** e.g. coryza, tonsillitis, bronchitis, pneumonia.

Breast
1. Cracked nipple.
2. Mastitis
   'Flushed breast'.
   Breast abscess.

Urinary Tract (a mid-stream specimen of urine will confirm the diagnosis)
1. Pyelitis.
2. Cystitis.

Phlebitis. *See below.*

THROMBO-EMBOLIC PHENOMENA

Types

Superficial Thrombophlebitis

1. *Pathology.* An infected clot in a superficial vein of the leg. The vein is usually the internal saphenous vein on the inside of the thigh, and is usually varicose.

2. *Clinically.* Pain and tenderness over the vein involved. An area of dull red induration surrounds the lesion. There may be pyrexia.

3. *Importance.* Does not usually lead to spread to the deep veins and to embolism but it may do so.

Deep Crural Phlebothrombosis

1. *Pathology.* A blood clot in a deep calf vein, usually in the soleus muscle. There is little surrounding inflammatory reaction, as a rule, so that the local symptoms and signs may be slight.

2. *Clinically*

a. Pain and tenderness over the calf with a positive Homan's sign.

b. Mild general reaction (e.g. a minor rise of pulse rate and temperature).

c. May be some swelling of the leg below the knee.

3. *Importance*

a. Embolism: bland clot moves more easily than an infected one.

b. Upward spread to produce a deep iliofemoral thrombophlebitis.

Deep Iliofemoral Thrombophlebitis

1. *Pathology*

a. An *infected clot* in the *iliofemoral vein* and its tributaries.

b. The infective process involves the *lymphatics* of the limb which follow the vein.

c. There is a *reflex spasm* of all vessels of the limb which:

Favours further extension of the clot.
Produces blanching and coldness of the leg,
especially the foot.
d. Oedema develops, as both vein and
lymphatic drainage are involved.
N.B. Simple venous obstruction, e.g. after
venous ligation, does not produce oedema, or
at least only a transitory one.
Its *extent* depends upon:
(1) The degree of involvement of the
lymphatics. (2) The number of collateral
channels involved. (3) The amount of
angiospasm present.
Its *persistence* depends upon:
(1) The extent to which there is irreversible
blockage—or reversible spasm. (2) The amount
of lymphatic involvement (marked lymphatic
blockage leads to a permanent non-pitting
oedema; venous blockage may be compensated
for by collateral circulation). (3) The extent to
which collateral channels have been blocked
or are capable of opening. (4) The degree of
valvular incompetence which results after
recanalization of a blocked vein. (5)
Ambulation in the early stages without
adequate support to the leg to reduce oedema.
*e. Chronic 'white leg' may develop
(phlegmasia alba dolens).* (1) Gross persistent
non-pitting oedema. (2) Trophic eczema and
ulceration.
The weight and discomfort of the leg is such
that it is a great burden to its possessor:
indeed, in severe cases even amputation might
be a relief.

2. *Clinically*
a. Pain and tenderness over Scarpa's triangle
and the external iliac vein.
b. There may be some initial blanching of the
leg and a cold foot.
c. Oedema of the whole leg may be mild or
gross. Daily measurements of the circumference
at different levels should be made and
recorded.

d. General reaction (e.g. pyrexia and raised pulse rate) may be absent or severe.

e. An ultrasound blood flow detector will show no signal over the vein in Scarpa's triangle when the calf is suddenly constricted.

3. *Importance*

a. The crippling, remote effects of the *chronic 'white leg'.*

b. Pulmonary embolism. Not so common as with the phlebothrombosis of the calf, for the infected clot is more fixed. It is probably newly formed clot, superimposed upon that already present, which shifts.

Embolism

1. *Pathology.* Clot breaks off from a venous thrombosis and moves through the right auricle and right ventricle to the pulmonary arteries and their branches. Its progress is arrested by the decreasing lumen of the pulmonary circulation, the level depending upon the size of the clot.

a. A large clot may block the main pulmonary artery with instant death.

b. A small clot may only block a terminal arteriole with the formation of a wedge-shaped infarct towards the periphery of the lung. There will be a patch of pleurisy on the outer surface.

2. *Clinically*

a. Severe cases—sudden death.

b. Mild cases—sudden onset of:

Pleural pain (pain on inspiration).

Dyspnoea and cyanosis (depending upon the extent of the lesion).

N.B. Search may or may not reveal the site of the primary thrombosis. *All pleural-type pain in the puerperium or after operation must be regarded as being due to pulmonary embolism and treated as such.*

Predisposi- tions

Recent Operation or Delivery

Thrombo-embolic phenomena tend to occur

most frequently about the 10th day after delivery or operation, due to certain *blood changes favouring coagulation* reaching their peak at this time. Other factors involved are listed below.

Blood Stasis due to Inactivity in Bed
Thrombosis and embolism can occur in the elderly even in medical cases.

Infection

Anaemia and Postpartum Haemorrhage

Tissue Damage at Operation

Age

History of Previous Thrombosis

Family History of Thrombosis and Varicose Veins

Sickle-cell Disease

Prophylaxis

1. Active movements after delivery and true early ambulation (*see* p. 207).
2. Avoidance and early treatment of sepsis.
3. Cure anaemia during pregnancy.
4. Careful operating with the minimum of trauma.

Treatment

Treatment in the Acute Phase of Thrombosis
1. Local heat by kaolin or heat cradle.
N.B. Glycerin and ichthyol is messy and no more effective than kaolin: it is unlikely that the ingredients are absorbed to produce any useful effect. Do not bandage the limb tightly so as to restrict movement.
2. Chemotherapy.
3. Active movements as soon as the relief from pain allows. Keep the bedclothes elevated by a cradle.
4. Ambulation as soon as possible (*see below*).

Paravertebral Sympathetic Block

1. *Use.* To block the sympathetic ganglia in the lumbar region which supply the autonomic nerves to the lower limbs. This abolishes the angiospasm which is present and:
a. Improves the circulation by:
(1) *Reducing oedema,* and
(2) Preventing *further spread of the clotting process.* New clot may: (i) Lead to *embolism.* (ii) Block further collaterals and lead to *permanent interference with the circulation.*
b. Reduces pain.
2. *Technique.* A trolley similar to that required for a spinal injection is required, but: A special needle at least 15 cm long is needed, and lignocaine (Xylocaine) 1%, or some other local anaesthetic is required.

Anticoagulants

1. *Use.* To *reduce the clotting power of the blood* after a thrombo-embolic incident, thereby preventing the deposition of further clot which might:
Lead to *embolism* or further embolism.
Block further collaterals leading to *permanent interference with the circulation.*
2. *Technique: Drugs Used. Heparin* (which acts at once but has to be given intravenously) and *warfarin* (which takes 24–36 hours to produce a therapeutic effect but can be given orally) are started simultaneously. Once the warfarin is acting the heparin is discontinued.
a. Heparin
Effective only *intravenously* (intramuscular heparin is not reliable).
DOSAGE: i.v. injection 100 mg (10000 units) lasts 4 hr. 150 mg (15000 units) lasts 6 hr.
or i.v. infusion 5000 units as a loading dose then 1500 units per hour.
The antidote is *protamine sulphate* injection but due to the short action of heparin it is seldom required. Dosage by slow i.v. injection,

if given within 15 min of the heparin administration, 15 mg of protamine to 1500 units of heparin given. The maximum dose is 50 mg.

Heparin acts by interfering with the actual fibrin formation.

b. Warfarin sodium

ROUTE   Orally.

DOSAGE   Initial loading dose of 40–50 mg. It takes 24–36 hours to produce a therapeutic level.

Subsequent dosage is governed by the daily prothrombin time, but most patients can be stabilized on a daily maintenance dose of between 3 and 10 mg.

Sensitivity to warfarin is increased by:
  Alcohol
  Chloramphenicol
  Cimetidine
  Co-trimoxazole
  Metronidazole
  Salicylates
  Sulphonamides
  Thyroxin

Therapy is continued so long as there is a danger of a further incident and in any case until the patient is fully ambulant. Breast feeding is not contraindicated.

PROTHROMBIN TIME A control estimation is made before therapy commences, e.g. if the control is 12 seconds:

Therapeutic level is 30 seconds (2½ times the control).

Therapeutic range is between 18 and 34 seconds.

No heparin should be given less than 12 or preferably 24 hours before performing the test, as the result may be invalidated.

4·5 ml of blood are put into a special bottle containing anticoagulant and shaken well to prevent clotting.

Warfarin therapy must never be undertaken without this control.

The *danger* is widespread spontaneous haemorrhage: haematuria is the earliest sign as a rule, and all specimens of urine must be examined with this in mind.

The *antidote* is *phytomenadione* (vitamin K_1) 5–20 mg i.v. (repeated if necessary in 2–3 hours) and transfusion with *fresh blood.*

Warfarin *acts on the liver,* preventing the production of prothrombin which is a vital component of the clotting process.

Scheme for Anticoagulant Therapy

	Time	Heparin	Warfarin	Prothrombin Time
1st day	10.00 hr	100 mg	40–50 mg	Specimen taken
	14.00 hr	100 mg		
	18.00 hr	150 mg		
	24.00 hr	150 mg		
2nd day	06.00 hr	100 mg		
	10.00 hr	100 mg		
	14.00 hr	100 mg		
	18.00 hr	150 mg		
	24.00 hr	None		
3rd day etc.	09.00 hr	(Only if		Specimen taken
	12.00 hr	required)	As required	Result received

Subsequent prothrombin times need to be performed:

On the 6th day	⎫ The laboratory will advise on
On the 9th day	⎪ the dose of warfarin when
After a further week	⎬ notifying the result of the
Thereafter only monthly	⎭ prothrombin time

Ligation of the Femoral Vein

1. *Use.* When recurrent sublethal pulmonary emboli are occurring despite anticoagulants. The indications are few and the operation is no longer popular.

2. *Technique.* The superficial femoral vein is ligated in Scarpa's triangle to prevent emboli escaping from the leg towards the heart.

N.B. It will fail if the emboli are arising from a higher level.

General Treatment for the Leg on Ambulation

1. The leg should be supported by an elastic bandage to reduce oedema while walking. This should be applied after elevating the leg until the oedema has been reduced as much as possible.

2. Massage helps to reduce oedema.

Pulmonary Embolism can only be treated symptomatically if the patient survives the initial incident.

1. Oxygen—if required.

2. Analgesics—for the pleural pain.

3. Antibiotics—to combat pneumonia.

At one time the title of this chapter would have been 'Prolonged Labour', but the emphasis has now shifted from considering the length of labour to observing the steady progress of labour, i.e. the continued dilatation of the cervix, the objects being to:

1. Accelerate labour as soon as it is clear that the *rate of cervical dilatation is falling below the norm,* and

2. Deliver the baby by Caesarean section when the attempt to accelerate labour has failed.

The only use for recording the total length of labour is to include in an Annual Obstetric Report those labours which have exceeded 24 hours.

CLASSIFICATION OF INEFFICIENT UTERINE ACTION (JEFFCOATE— MODIFIED)

Hypotonic Inertia

1. Soft uterus between contractions.
2. Feeble uterine contractions, but with normal fundal dominance.
3. The mother is not at all distressed by the contractions.

Hypertonic 'Inertia' (Inco-ordinate Uterine Action—a Better Term)	**1.** Uterus is hard between contractions. **2.** The uterus may be contracting quite strongly but is ineffective in dilating the cervix as fundal dominance is absent. **3.** The mother is quite distressed by the pains and is, in addition, worn down by the continuous ache between contractions. This ache may be abdominal but is usually midsacral.

SPECIAL TYPES OF INCOORDINATE UTERUS

Hypertonic Lower Uterine Segment	**1.** Thick, resistant lower uterine segment which does not dilate. **2.** Severe midsacral backache.
'Colicky Uterus'	**1.** Irregular painful contractions with slow dilatation of the cervix. **2.** Continuous ache in the hypogastrium.
Generally Contracted Uterus	**1.** The whole uterus is moulding itself round the baby. In its extreme form the presenting part may even be lifted out of the pelvis. **2.** Fetal distress is imminent in this type of case.
Constriction or Contraction Ring	**1.** A *localized spasm* of a ring of uterine muscle, actively holding the baby in the uterus. It usually occurs at the physiological retraction ring but may occur elsewhere in the uterus. **2.** During a contraction the presenting part becomes freer instead of being pressed into the pelvis. **3.** It is a potentially *reversible condition* which may well occur before full dilatation.

N.B. It must be distinguished from *pathological retraction ring* (or *Bandl's ring*), which occurs as a result of obstructed labour and always after full dilatation has been reached. It is not reversible until the baby is delivered.

False Labour

This is a form of incoordinate uterine action, which differs from an incoordinate true labour only in that the *cervix has not yet begun to dilate.*

It may be regarded as an exaggerated form of the 'painless' contractions of Braxton-Hicks, which, indeed, are often not painless.

False labour may:

1. Pass off altogether; true labour will begin at some later date.

2. Change suddenly into true efficient labour.

3. Merge imperceptibly into true, but inefficient labour, i.e. the cervix will begin to dilate, slowly and tediously.

PRIMARY OR SECONDARY UTERINE INERTIA

This is another method of classification. It implies either that the condition is there from the outset, or develops in the course of the labour. This classification has, however, little clinical significance, while being a useful descriptive nomenclature.

Referring to 'secondary inertia' as resulting from an 'exhausted uterus' is, however, rather more a poetic analogy than an aetiological concept based on sound evidence.

CAUSE

The cause of inefficient uterine action is unknown.

Associated Factors

Primigravid Patients are most commonly affected; inefficient uterine action is rare after vaginal delivery has been affected once.

High Presenting Part in the Primigravid Case is frequently associated with inefficient uterine action.

Theory of Bipolarity

This postulates that pressure by the presenting part on the lower segment stimulates by reflex the upper segment to contract. If the presenting part is high this mechanism is absent. But why then is inefficient uterine action so seldom present in multiparous women when the presenting part is usually high at term? The evidence for the existence of a bipolarity mechanism is rather unconvincing.

Causes of High Head at Term in the Primigravid Case:

1. Posterior positions of the occiput.
2. Abnormal pelvid shape favouring posterior position:
a. Android
b. Anthropoid } brim.
3. Disproportion.

Fear or Other Unfavourable Mental Attitude leads to inertia—and this is the basis of the theories of Grantly Dick-Read. Young girls with suppressed fears, or women who know that the baby has died in utero, are examples of cases which labour badly.

Factors of Doubtful Importance

Age

General Debility and Anaemia
Such patients, however, stand prolonged labour ill.

Reflex Inhibition of Uterine Action by Full Bladder or Loaded Rectum
It is more likely that the inactivity of these viscera results from the same cause as that causing the uterine aberration (Jeffcoate).

Factors not Responsible for Uterine Inefficiency

Over-distension of the Uterus, e.g. twins and polyhydramnios (Jeffcoate). However, postpartum haemorrhage *is* a sequel to these conditions, and some people regard this as inefficient uterine action in the third stage.

Rupture of Membranes, if anything, accelerates labour rather than the opposite, all things being equal. However:
1. Premature rupture of the membranes may be due to other conditions which are associated with inefficient uterine action, e.g. posterior position, android pelvis, etc.
2. It is stressed that membranes rupturing early in the course of a prolonged labour is of bad prognosis.

DANGERS

To the Mother

1. *Sepsis.*
2. *Exhaustion.*
3. *Postpartum Haemorrhage.*
4. *Morbidity* or even death due to *obstetrical interference* (e.g. Caesarean section, forceps, etc.) in a patient whose condition may already be poor as a result of a long labour.
5. *Inhalation Pneumonia* as a result of food being retained in the stomach for long periods of time; another example of smooth muscle inefficiency accompanying abnormal uterine action.
Maternal deaths from this cause are remaining alarmingly frequent.
Precautions:
a. Avoid general anaesthesia whenever possible by the use of pudendal block.
b. Obstetric anaesthesia requires a skilled anaesthetist with intubation and suction facilities available.
c. Give only fluids in labour.
d. Before inducing anaesthesia: (1) A gastric tube must be passed. (2) Mist. Mag. Trisil. 15 ml is given.

(In all cases in late pregnancy whether 'starved' or not.)

6. *Annular Detachment of the Cervix.*

To the Baby

1. *Asphyxia* due to interference with the placental circulation, particularly with high-tone 'inertia'. The baby is much safer with low-tone inertia and if the membranes are intact.

2. *Birth Injury* following a difficult forceps extraction.

3. *Neonatal Pneumonia* due to intra-uterine infection after rupture of the membranes.

MANAGEMENT

Determine the Time of Onset of True Labour

I.e. when cervical dilatation and regular contractions begin. 'False labour' is best treated by sedation and reassurance that she is not yet in labour.

General Measures

1. Intravenous glucose-saline may be necessary if ketonuria develops, but do not immobilize the patient with a 'drip' until it is required.

2. Sleep and sedation. Epidural analgesia is an important element in the management of inefficient uterine actions.

3. Reassurance.

4. Walking about may stimulate contractions and improve the patient's outlook if she is not immobilized by sedation, a 'drip', or a monitor.

Observations which Determine Further Management

Maternal Condition

1. Pulse.

2. Temperature.

3. Urine ketones.

4. Fluid balance.

5. General condition and mental state.

Fetal Condition
1. Fetal heart rate and regularity (*see* Fetal Monitoring, p. 187).
2. Presence or absence of meconium.

Progress of the Labour
1. Frequency and strength of contractions.
2. Membranes—intact or ruptured.
3. Cervix:
a. Dilating.
b. Thinning or becoming thicker.
c. Applied or not.
4. Presenting part:
a. Descending.
b. Moulding.
c. Rotating (if posterior position).

Decision to Continue the Labour

1. The dilatation of the cervix must be assessed approximately every 3 hours, preferably by the same person. If this is not possible there should be a careful 'hand-over' from one observer to the next. It must be stressed that *steady dilatation of the cervix is the only index of the progress of labour.* The descent of the head, for example, has very little importance in this context despite much teaching to the contrary.
2. Once the cervix has begun to dilate (i.e. true labour has begun), if after a 3-hour interval, and certainly after a 6-hour interval, the dilatation of the cervix has been slow or absent, *the membranes should be ruptured* (if still intact), and the *labour accelerated by oxytocin* (*see below*).
3. If after 6 hours on oxytocin there has been no change in the cervical dilatation, serious consideration must be given to delivering the baby by *Caesarean section.*
N.B. At each 3-hourly assessment all the factors referred to under Observations which determine Further Management must be taken into account and the questions asked:
a. Is it safe to mother and baby to continue with the labour? and

b. If the labour does go on, is vaginal delivery likely to be achieved while it still is safe?

If the answer to either question is 'No', then labour should be terminated forthwith.

Methods of Terminating Labour before Full Dilatation

1. Caesarean section.
2. Incision or dilatation of cervix and forceps delivery.
3. Vacuum extraction.

Some Special Methods of Management

Intravenous Infusion of Oxytocin (supplied in its synthetic form, Syntocinon)

1. *Types of Case*

Failure of the labour to progress (*see above*) is now considered the only indication for accelerating labour although at one time it was considered that cases of incoordinate uterine action might not respond; perhaps the success rate may be less in such cases but it is worth trying. O'Driscoll (1969)* was one of the pioneers of augmenting labour.

Considerable caution is required in certain cases:

a. Those with a history of previous Caesarean section (some would never use oxytocin in these cases).

b. 'Grand multips'.

c. Cases of disproportion, especially in the late first stage, and when the head is no longer easily displaced upwards: at this stage the lower segment is becoming stressed.

2. *Method*

a. Simple 'drip' (an automatic drip counter is an advantage).

Oxytocin 1 unit/500 ml of dextrose.

Start at 10 drops/min.

Increase every 30 min by 10 drops/min until

*O'Driscoll K., Jackson R. J. A., and Gallagher J. T. (1969) *Br. Med. J.* **2**, 477–480

60 drops/min is reached (approximately 8 mu/min).
Replace the original solution with 2 units/500 ml. Start at 30 drops/min and increase as before until 60 drops/min is reached.
N.B.   Increase beyond 8 mu/min requires careful consideration.
b. 'Cardiff' infusor.
Oxytocin 10 units/500 ml of dextrose.
The machine increases the dose automatically from 1 to 32 mu/min over 75 min.
3. *Dangers*
a. Rupture of uterus.
N.B.   Contractions must be watched constantly and if they become severe, the drip must be cut back at once.
b. Death of fetus due to interference with placental circulation.
4. *Observations*
Keep a careful partograph and use continuous fetal monitoring.
5. *Continuation of oxytocic drip* until well after delivery of the placenta is required. Premature interruption may produce the following according to the stage when the drip is stopped:
a. Delay in 2nd stage requiring forceps.
b. Retained placenta.
c. PPH.

Epidural Anaesthesia in cases of incoordinate uterine action may speed up progress to full dilatation. In any case it is of particular help in these cases for relief of the persistent pain even if the technique is not being used routinely on normal labours.

Constriction Ring
1. Sedate and await relaxation—no immediate danger.
2. Relax the ring by:

| Deep anaesthesia, or | If delivery is |
| Amyl nitrite | essential. |

3. Occasionally Caesarean section may be required.

PROGNOSIS FOR FUTURE LABOURS

1. A primigravida who has had a vaginal delivery can safely be reassured that a recurrence of prolonged labour in future is unlikely.

2. If the outcome was by Caesarean section, it is still possible to get a normal labour next time, but there is more chance of a repeated inefficient uterine action than if vaginal delivery had occurred.

If the cervix reached half dilatation or more before Caesarean section was performed, the prognosis for vaginal delivery next time is reasonably good.

Precipitate Labour

DEFINITION

Delivery of the baby within such a short period of time that the mother had almost no warning.

FACTORS INVOLVED

1. Lack of resistance from the maternal soft parts.
2. Powerful, prolonged and frequent uterine contractions.

INCIDENCE

It is an uncommon event and is usually due to the lack of resistance by the maternal soft parts.

DANGERS

Fetal

Trauma by Falling, if the mother is caught unawares, e.g. standing or on the toilet. (The baby is not likely to suffer cerebral damage by rapid passage through the pelvis and soft tissues, if it is the lack of resistance by the latter rather than the force driving the baby which is the main factor: there is a popular confusion of thought concerning this.)

Cerebral Damage may occur if the baby is forced out by powerful contractions against normal or nearly normal soft-tissue resistance.

Maternal

1. *Rupture of uterus* (if the contractions are violent).
2. Severe *vulval laceration.*

25 Disproportion

LEVELS AT WHICH DISPROPORTION CAN OCCUR

1. Brim.
2. Plane of least dimensions.
3. Outlet.
As it is extremely rare for insuperable disproportion to arise once the head has passed the brim, more attention is paid to the brim level than any other. This is fortunate, because:
1. The brim is easier to measure than the other levels.
2. The relationship between head and brim can be tested before labour begins.

MECHANISMS BY WHICH DISPROPORTION IS OVERCOME

Moulding of the fetal skull.

Asynclitism (anterior parietal presentation is the most favourable). This mechanism allows the *sub-supraparietal diameter* of 8·0 cm to engage the anteroposterior diameter of the brim instead of the *biparietal* of 9·5 cm.

Sideways Displacement of the head in rachitic pelvis which has a wide transverse diameter of the brim. This allows the bitemporal diameter to engage the brim.

DIAGNOSIS OF CONTRACTED PELVIS

(Assuming a normal vertex presentation). All cases (multiparae or primigravidae) should have the pelvis assessed by a doctor at 36 weeks' gestation, particularly if home confinement is contemplated, proceeding as follows:

1. If the *fetal is already engaged* there will be no disproportion at full term.

2. If the head is not engaged, *head fitting* will be undertaken by one of the following methods:

a. With the patient on her back, press the head down in the axis of the pelvis, or

b. With the patient sitting, but leaning back on her arm, see if the head has entered the brim, or

c. With the patient erect, but leaning forward on outstretched arms, palpate to see if the head is engaged.

3. If head fitting cannot be achieved, either because of soft tissue resistance or bony disproportion, the pelvis should be estimated by *vaginal examination.* Note should be made of:

a. The *diagonal conjugate.* The *internal conjugate* is estimated by subtracting 1·5 cm from the diagonal conjugate, i.e. the pelvis can only be taken as adequate if the diagonal conjugate equals or exceeds 12·5 cm.

b. The prominence of the *ischial spines.*

c. The curve of the *sacrum.*

d. The *anteroposterior diameter of the plane of least dimensions.*

e. The shape and width of the *pubic arch.*

4. If the vaginal examination is unsatisfactory

because the soft tissue resistance prevents the obstetrician from reaching at least 12·5 cm, *X-ray pelvimetry* should be employed.
N.B.   Contracted pelvis cannot be excluded on a history of previous vaginal vertex deliveries whatever the weights of the babies.

MANAGEMENT

N.B.   Always confine in a specialist unit.

Trial of Labour

Special Points
1. The vertex must be presenting.
2. Onset of labour must be spontaneous, or, at the most, induced medically (surgical induction is contra-indicated).
3. Strictly speaking the term 'trial of labour' is restricted to the case in her first labour.

Observations and Management are as under 'Inefficient Uterine Action' (q.v.). Where a trial of labour fails to achieve vaginal delivery it is usually because of the associated inefficient uterine action, not the disproportion itself.

Method of Terminating
1. Spontaneous delivery.
2. Forceps delivery or vacuum extraction.
3. Caesarean section.

Elective Caesarean

Definition
Delivery of the baby, abdominally, before the onset of labour as a planned policy—usually at 38 or 39 weeks.

Indications
N.B.   It is almost never required with disproportion as the *only* indication, but it may be indicated as follows:
1. *Previous Caesarean section* after an adequate trial of labour.

2. Marked disproportion in an *elderly primigravida.*
3. *Breech presentation* with contracted pelvis.

Induction of Premature Labour

Technique
Surgical induction of labour by artificial rupture of the membranes to get a smaller baby with a more mouldable head.

Indications (very rarely done nowadays and has never been popular outside the British Isles). A *multiparous* patient in whom it was considered that a previous delivery had only just succeeded.

Period of Gestation
Not under 38 weeks.

Postpartum Haemorrhage including Third-stage Haemorrhage

DEFINITIONS

Postpartum Haemorrhage

A loss of 500 ml or more after delivery of the child. It can, however, be subdivided into:
1. *Third-stage Haemorrhage* (bleeding while the placenta is still in situ).
2. *True Postpartum Haemorrhage* (after the third stage is completed).
If not otherwise stated, always assume that '*postpartum haemorrhage*' includes 'third-stage haemorrhage'.
N.B. Blood loss must be considered abnormal and action taken long before 500 ml is lost.

Causes *See below.*

Delayed Postpartum Haemorrhage

A loss occurring over one hour and under 24 hours after delivery of the placenta.

Causes
1. Retained products of conception.
2. Blood clot.

Secondary Postpartum Haemorrhage

A loss occurring after the first 24 hours from delivery of the placenta: it may occur weeks later.

Causes
1. Retained products of conception.
2. Sepsis.
3. Hormonal. In most cases of secondary postpartum haemorrhage no residual pregnancy material is found in the uterus; such bleeding is probably due to the changes which are occurring in the hormonal balance while the system is returning to its normal periodicity.

CAUSES OF POSTPARTUM HAEMORRHAGE

From the Placental Site

Imperfect Uterine Retraction due to the Uterus not being Empty
1. Partial separation of the placenta. A localized patch of placenta accreta may occur. The placenta may be adherent to the scar of a previous Caesarean section.
2. Retained placental tissue, e.g. a cotyledon or a succenturiate lobe.
3. Blood clot—perhaps through inadequate attention to the height of the fundus after delivery of the placenta: a vicious circle, for clot leads to bleeding which leads to more clot.

Atony of the Uterus associated with:
1. Inefficient uterine action in the 1st and 2nd stages.
2. Overdistension of the uterus:

a. Twins ⎫ These do not necessarily lead to inefficient uterine
b. Polyhydramnios ⎭ action in the 1st and 2nd stages.

3. Grand multiparity.
4. Fibroids.

Sepsis
Causes separation of the clot sealing a uterine sinus: leads to secondary postpartum haemorrhage.

Clotting Defect (*see* details of coagulation and fibrinolysis mechanisms, *Tables* 2, 3, pp. 246, 247).

1. *Fetal Death in Utero* for 3 weeks or more.

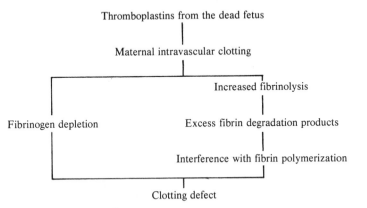

Thromboplastins from the dead fetus

Maternal intravascular clotting

Increased fibrinolysis

Fibrinogen depletion

Excess fibrin degradation products

Interference with fibrin polymerization

Clotting defect

2. *Severe Concealed Accidental Haemorrhage.* Thromboplastins for the damaged placenta act as in Fetal Death in Utero.

3. *Amniotic Embolism*

a. Timing: When the membranes rupture, especially with strong contractions.

b. Pathology: Some constituent of the amniotic fluid enters the maternal circulation and causes:

a. Disseminated intravascular coagulation which leads to: (i) Clotting defect (as for Fetal Death in Utero—*see above*). (ii) Thrombosis in pulmonary vessels.

b. Anaphylactic shock.

c. At postmortem examination, fetal squames are found in the pulmonary capillaries.

Clinically

a. Severe shock.

b. Respiratory distress and cyanosis (X-ray of the chest shows widespread opacities).

c. Postpartum haemorrhage.

d. Death is common.

4. *Septic Abortion*
Pathology: Endotoxins enter the maternal circulation and cause:
a. Bacteriaemic shock.
b. Intravascular clotting which leads to: (i) Clotting defect (as in 1 above). (ii) Micro-embolism in renal capillaries.
Clinically
a. Profound shock.
b. Temperature may be raised or low.
c. Heavy uterine bleeding.
d. Anuria.

Traumatic

1. A tear of cervix, vagina, or vulva. May follow spontaneous or instrumental delivery.
2. Rupture of a varicose vein of the vulva.

N.B.   Many cases of postpartum haemorrhage occur where no obvious cause is found, but recurrence of postpartum haemorrhage (as well as retained placenta) in succeeding labours is very common.

TREATMENT

Prophylaxis

1. Anticipate the cases in which haemorrhage is likely, i.e. the cases listed as being liable to atony of the uterus in the third stage and also patients with a history of a previous postpartum haemorrhage.
a. Confine these cases in hospital.
b. Have a doctor present at delivery.
c. Give ergometrine intravenously after delivering the anterior shoulder of the baby.
2. Watch the fundus when the placenta is out to prevent blood clot collecting unnoticed.

Bleeding from the Placental Site—Shock not Present

Rub up a Contraction and expel blood clot.

Ergometrine intravenously and intramuscularly —0·25 mg by each route, whether the placenta is in or out of the uterus. If bleeding continues it may be advisable to give oxytocin 5 units as an alternative to repeating ergometrine. Attempt, periodically, to deliver the placenta by controlled cord traction, so long as the uterus is firmly contracted.

A Midwife should send for Medical Aid

Placenta still in Utero

1. *Repeat Controlled Cord Traction*
2. *Manual Removal of the Placenta.* An anaesthetic is used, but in an emergency it can be done without; the midwife should not attempt it unless completely cut off from help. The manoeuvre should be done early, before the blood loss is serious.

Placenta out and Bleeding Continuing

1. *First Consider*
a. Traumatic bleeding (*see below*).
b. Clotting Defect
  i. Prolonged fetal death in utero
  ii. Severe concealed accidental haemorrhage *see* p. 113.
  iii. Amniotic embolism
    As the pulmonary aspect predominates in amniotic embolism, heparin is advocated and antifibrinolytic therapy is deprecated.
  iv. Septic abortion.
    Antibiotics and evacuation of uterus.
    Blood and fibrinogen.
    Antifibrinolytic therapy may prejudice the kidney function.
    Heparin is probably useless at the best and may make matters worse.
2. *Explore the Uterus* to remove placental residue and clot (if not already done).
3. *Bimanual Compression*
a. An emergency method for severe bleeding.

b. The right fist is placed in the anterior fornix and the uterus dragged over it and the pubis by the left hand on the abdomen. It is maintained until the uterus is felt to regain tone.

4. *Hot Intra-uterine Douche*
a. Temperature 48°C—a douche can, rubber tube and nozzle will be required.
b. Given under anaesthetic after manual removal.

5. *Intra-uterine Pack*
a. Several rolls of sterile 15 cm gauze may be required.
b. Performed under anaesthesia, packing right to the fundus.

6. *Compression of the Aorta* against the lumbar spine through the anterior abdominal wall. Only likely to succeed in thin patients.

7. *Hysterectomy* as a last resort.

Bleeding from the Placental Site— Patient Shocked

Clinically
The bleeding will usually have stopped due to the low blood pressure.

Action by the Midwife
1. Send for medical aid (patient's doctor or the Flying Squad) and give the blood group.
2. Give ergometrine.
3. When the uterus contracts, expel blood clot and the placenta, if it is in the vagina.
N.B. On no account attempt further controlled cord traction.
4. Keep the patient dry and give mouthwashes but nothing to drink in case an anaesthetic is required.
N.B. Elevation of the foot of the bed is of doubtful value unless very high and then it is most uncomfortable: it is better not to do it.
5. Prepare for manual removal of the placenta.

Action by the Doctor
1. Start a blood drip.

2. If the placenta is out, perform a vaginal examination gently to exclude:
a. Acute inversion of the uterus.
b. A piece of placenta lying in the cervix.
3. When the patient begins to recover or if bleeding begins again, proceed as *above,* Placenta still in Utero, or Placenta out and Bleeding Continuing.

Traumatic Bleeding

(Bleeding continues despite a contracted fundus)

Vulval or Vaginal Lacerations
Control bleeding by:
1. Pressure with gauze—immediately.
2. Suture or ligature—as soon as possible.

Cervical Lacerations
Apply sponge-holding forceps to both lips of the cervix and draw it down for inspection, using vaginal retractions. Suture the laceration, beginning at the apex of the tear.

Tears into the Parametrium
1. Pack with 15 cm gauze, or
2. Laparotomy to find the bleeding artery (not easy).

Delayed Postpartum Bleeding

(Retained placental tissue or clot)
1. Resuscitate if necessary.
2. Give ergometrine and expel vaginal clot.
3. Explore the uterus digitally if bleeding continues.

Secondary Postpartum Bleeding

(Retained placental tissue or sepsis) As in Delayed Postpartum Bleeding, but the blunt Rheinstätter curette may be needed.

COAGULATION AND FIBRINOLYSIS MECHANISMS

Factors Involved which are Normal Constituents of Plasma

A. COAGULATION		B. FIBRINOLYSIS
1. *Activating*		1. *Activating*

		Plasminogen
Factor XIII	Fibrin stabilizing factor	
Factor XII	Hageman factor	
Factor XI	Plasma thromboplastin antecedent	
Factor X	Stuart–Prower factor	
Factor IX	Christmas factor	
Factor VIII	Antihaemophilic globulin	
Factor VII	Stable factor	
Factor V	Labile factor	
Factor IV	Calcium	
Factor II	Prothrombin	
Factor I	Fibrinogens	

2. *Inhibitory*

Antithrombin

2. *Inhibitory*

Antiplasmin

N.B. Thromboplastin (Factor III) is not a single entity (*see Tables* 2 *and* 3, pp. 246 and 247)

Factors Involved which Initiate the Processes

Processes involved	Activators
Activation of Factors XI and XII	A variety of non-specific agents both extrinsic from damaged tissue or intrinsic from damaged vessels.
Activation of Factor X	Phospholipids from damaged tissues (extrinsic) or from damaged platelets (intrinsic). (Along with other factors (*see Table* 2))
Conversion of prothrombin to thrombin	Phospholipids from damaged tissue and platelets (as part of the thromboplastin complex)
Plasminogen activation	A variety of agents

(*See Tables* 2 *and* 3, pp. 246 and 247.)

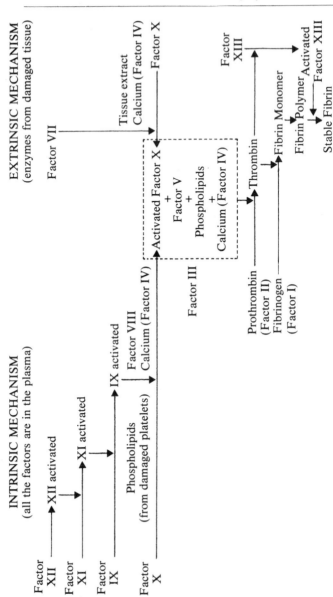

Table 2. Initiation of coagulation

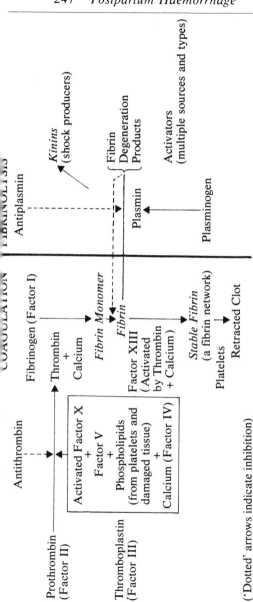

Table 3. Coagulation and fibrinolysis mechanisms

27 Posterior Position of the Occiput

FAVOURED BY

1. Android and anthropoid pelvic brims.
2. Brims with steep angle of inclination.

MECHANISM

Long Internal Rotation

(90% of occipitoposterior positions)

Descent

Flexion
Imperfect: suboccipitofrontal diameter presents (10 cm) but later flexes until the suboccipito-bregmatic diameter presents (9·5 cm).

Internal Rotation
Three-eighths of a circle. Occiput meets the pelvic gutter first.
   At this stage the shoulders may either remain in the same oblique, maintaining a three-eighths of a circle twist on the neck, or else the posterior shoulder may cross the midline which reduces the twist on the neck to one-eighth of a circle.

Extension
To allow the birth of the head.

First Mechanism	*Second Mechanism*
(Shoulders do not move)	*(Shoulders move)*
Restitution	
Three-eighths of a circle: opposite direction to internal rotation	One-eighth of a circle: opposite direction to internal rotation
External Rotation	
One-eighth of a circle: same direction as internal rotation	One-eighth of a circle: opposite direction to internal rotation

Lateral Flexion

N.B. In either mechanism the head is born as in a normal anterior position of the vertex and in the second mechanism the whole procedure from extension onwards follows the course of events as in a normal vertex delivery with the occiput anterior.

Short Internal Rotation

(10% of occipitoposterior positions)

Descent

Flexion
Very imperfect: occipitofrontal diameter presents (11·5 cm) and fails to flex further.

Internal Rotation
One-eighth of a circle. Sinciput meets the pelvic gutter first and rotates forwards under the pubic arch.

Increased Flexion followed by Extension
Face-to-pubes delivery. The frontal region comes into contact with the pubis so that continued descent causes the head to flex and the occiput to escape over the perineum: after this the head falls back and the face wheels out from under the pubis.

Restitution
One-eighth of a circle (opposite direction to internal rotation).

External Rotation
As 'Restitution'.

Lateral Flexion

REASON FOR THE EXTENDED ATTITUDES

The convexity of the fetal spine lies against the convexity of the maternal spine which favours extension of the former.

DIAMETERS INVOLVED AT THE VULVA
(*see* p. 168)

Long Internal Rotation

Suboccipitofrontal (10 cm) and the bitemporal (8 cm) distend the vulva, as with an anterior position of the vertex.

Short Internal Rotation

(Face-to-pubes delivery): Occipitofrontal (11·5 cm) and the biparietal (9·5 cm) distend the vulva, i.e. 1·5 cm larger in each direction than with the long internal rotation.

EFFECT ON LABOUR

Prolonged First Stage due to Inefficient Uterine Action

The larger diameters interfere with descent of the head and therefore with pressure on the lower uterine segment. This reduces the effect of the hypothetical mechanism of 'bipolarity'.

The dangers to mother and baby are listed under 'Prolonged Labour', Chapter 23, but the result is *a higher maternal and fetal morbidity and mortality.*

Early Rupture of Membranes

The head does not fit the brim so well. It leads to:

Intra-uterine Sepsis

Fetal Death during Labour

Prolapsed Cord

Short Internal Rotation

(Persistent occipitoposterior or 'face-to-pubes' presentation).
1. 'Fading' of contractions in the second stage even if they had been good until then.
2. Delay in delivery of the head on the perineum despite reasonably good contractions and maternal effort.
3. Greater damage to perineum due to larger diameters.

DIAGNOSIS

Abdominally

1. Concavity of abdominal outline below the umbilicus.
2. High head in a primigravida at term.
3. Palpation of back difficult and limbs lie on both sides of abdomen.
4. Fetal heart is heard either right out in the flank or in the midline.

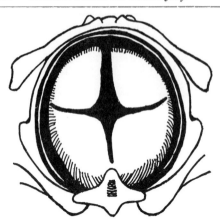

Fig. 15. Persistent occipitoposterior position or face-to-pubes (touch picture).

Vaginally	Palpation of sutures (*Fig.* 15).
By the Course of Labour	**1.** Inefficient uterine action in first stage. **2.** Delay in second stage or in delivery of head (*see* Short Internal Rotation, *above*).

OUTCOME AND MANAGEMENT

Long Internal Rotation and Spontaneous or Forceps Delivery

Deep Transverse Arrest

1. The head has failed to flex adequately and is found at the level of the spines with both fontanelles equally palpable: as there is equal pressure on both sides of the head further rotation is impossible.

2. May rise from:

a. A head which has entered the brim in the *occipitolateral position* and descended to the spines in that position.

b. An *occipitoposterior position* which has

begun to rotate but extension of the head and poor contractions caused the movement to halt.

3. It is favoured by:

a. A straight sacrum.

b. Prominent ischial spines.

c. Poor contractions.

4. *Treatment*

a. Manual rotation and forceps delivery, or

b. Rotation and delivery by Kielland's forceps.

Short Internal Rotation with:

1. *Face-to-pubes Delivery*

a. Spontaneous. Deep episiotomy is advisable on account of the severe vulval distension, or

b. Forceps. There is a tendency for the forceps to slip off.

2. *Occipito-anterior Delivery after:*

a. Manual rotation and forceps delivery, or

b. Rotation and delivery by Kielland's forceps.

Caesarean Section

1. Failure to progress in first stage.

2. Maternal or fetal distress.

Dead Baby and Prolonged First Stage

Craniotomy

28 Face Presentation

ORIGIN

Possibly by further extension of a posterior position of the occiput, the biparietal diameter of the fetal skull being trapped in the sacrocotyloid diameter (q.v.), but recent radiographic evidence tends to show that face presentation often develops before labour begins, not during labour.

Thyroid tumours and anencephaly favour face presentation.

POSITIONS

1st position RMP (from an LOA).
2nd position LMP (from an ROA).
3rd position LMA (from an ROP).
4th position RMA (from an LOP).
Nevertheless the order of frequency is LMA, RMA, RMP, LMP, i.e. it follows the same rules as for vertex presentation.

MECHANISM

Mento-anterior Positions

1. *Descent*
2. *Extension* (the submentobregmatic diameter of 9·5 cm presents).
3. *Internal Rotation* of one-eighth of a circle.
4. *Flexion*—to allow birth of the head.
5. *Restitution*—one-eighth of a circle in the opposite direction to internal rotation.
6. *External Rotation*—one-eighth of a circle in the opposite direction to internal rotation.
7. *Lateral Flexion.*

Mento-posterior Positions

Long Internal Rotation (this is unlikely to occur as the head is not pressing on the pelvic floor)

1. *Descent*
2. *Extension*
3. *Internal Rotation* of three-eighths of a circle. (Posterior shoulder may or may not cross the midline.)
4. *Flexion*
5. *Restitution.* One-eighth or three-eighths of a circle (in opposite direction to internal rotation)—cf. posterior position of occiput mechanism q.v.
6. *External Rotation.* One-eighth of a circle (either in the same or opposite direction to internal rotation).

Short Internal Rotation

1. *Descent*
2. *Extension*
3. *Internal Rotation* of one-eighth of a circle.
4. *Obstructed Labour.* This is because the head and the trunk try to enter the pelvic brim at the same time and this is impossible.

DIAMETERS INVOLVED AT THE VULVA

Submentovertical (11·5 cm) and the biparietal

(9·5 cm) distend the vulva—cf. 'Face-to-pubes' delivery (pp. 168 and 250).

DIAGNOSIS

Abdominally

1. Cephalic prominence on same side as the back.
2. Deep groove between occiput and back.

Vaginally

1. An irregular presenting part in which eventually the hard gums give a clue to the diagnosis.
2. The chin must be palpated to identify the position.

MANAGEMENT

A midwife should seek medical aid unless spontaneous delivery is imminent.

Mento-anterior and Mento-lateral Positions

1. Spontaneous delivery—usually requires an episiotomy.
2. Forceps delivery.

Mento-posterior Positions

1. Spontaneous rotation and delivery.
2. Manual rotation and forceps delivery, or Kielland's forceps rotation and extraction, e.g. after deep transverse arrest.
3. Conversion to vertex presentation and allow labour to continue (for persistent mentoposterior).
4. Occasionally Caesarean section is advisable.
N.B. Warn the mother before the baby is born that on account of the caput on the baby's face it will look rather repulsive at

birth, but that after three days at the most it will look quite normal.

EFFECT ON LABOUR

1. More traumatic to mother and baby than vertex presentation.
a. Danger of impaction, especially with mentoposterior position.
b. Wider diameters distending the vulva.
2. Premature rupture of membranes more likely than with vertex presentation.

29

Brow Presentation

MECHANISM

None. Occasionally a small baby may deliver spontaneously but this must never be expected.

DIAGNOSIS

By palpation of the *supra-orbital ridges* vaginally (*Fig.* 16).
1. An accidental finding.
2. Failure of the head to descend prompts a vaginal examination.
3. A wide head palpated abdominally leads to further investigation.

MANAGEMENT

1. Caesarean section—best treatment for the primigravid patient.
2. Convert to face or vertex and extract by forceps
3. Internal version and breech extraction
} Occasionally in multiparous patients
4. Craniotomy if the baby be dead.

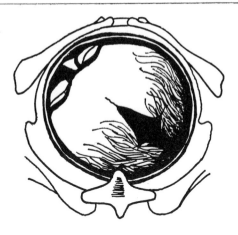

Fig. 16. Brow presentation (touch picture).

30

Transverse Lie

CAUSES

Factors preventing Part entering the Brim

1. Disproportion.
   a. Contracted pelvis.
   b. Hydrocephalus.
2. Masses in the pelvis.
   a. Fibroid.
   b. Ovarian tumour.
   c. Tumour of the pelvis.
   d. Non-pregnant horn of a uterus bicornis.
3. Placenta praevia.
4. Twins.

Factors allowing Undue Mobility of the Fetus

1. Polyhydramnios.
2. 'Grand' multiparity.
3. Prematurity.

Cordate Uterus

(Uterus subseptus)
The small septum interferes with longitudinal lie.

POSSIBLE PRESENTING PARTS

1. Shoulder.
2. Hand.
3. Elbow.

DANGERS

1. Premature rupture of membranes with prolapsed cord.
2. Obstructed labour with:
a. Death of the baby; and
b. Rupture of the uterus and death of the mother from shock and haemorrhage.

DIAGNOSIS

1. Abdominal examination (inspection and palpation).
2. Vaginal examination.
a. Shoulder presentation—distinguish from breech, face, or brow by palpation of the ribs.
b. Hand presentation—distinguish from a foot by the absence of a heel.
c. Elbow presentation—distinguish from a knee by feeling higher for the ribs or the hand.

MANAGEMENT

Pregnancy Under 38 Weeks but 34 Weeks or Over

N.B. Ask yourself, 'Why should there be a transverse lie?' Proceed as follows:
1. Ask if there has been any vaginal bleeding.
2. Perform external version.
3. Attempt to push the head into the pelvis. If this is not possible,
4. Perform a vaginal examination, unless the head is so high as to suggest a major degree of placenta praevia, when ultrasonography should be performed to exclude this.

5. Allow her to go home from the clinic, to return in one week.
6. Correct the lie each week so long as is necessary and the period of gestation is under 38 weeks.

Pregnancy 38 Weeks or Over

(Unstable lie)

Admit to hospital to await labour, correcting the lie from time to time.

N.B. Rupture of the forewaters with application of a binder has been advocated but in practice is an unsatisfactory treatment: the transverse lie usually recurs under the binder and now there would be ruptured membranes as well—a dangerous situation.

Recently an attempt to revive active treatment has been made. An oxytocic drip is set up and when contractions occur the forewaters are ruptured: it is claimed that under these circumstances the presenting part 'fixes'. Some people still have reservations concerning the safety of this procedure but it might be useful if postmaturity has become a superadded problem.

During Labour

Possible lines of treatment are:

a. External Version—so long as there is sufficient liquor, even if membranes are ruptured, but beware of prolapse of the cord.

b. Caesarean Section—safest for the baby: the only method if there is little or no liquor left.

c. Bipolar Podalic Version, or Internal Version—bringing down a leg and awaiting breech delivery—dangerous to the baby.

d. Internal Version and Breech Extraction—suitable for multiparous cases near full dilatation but with adequate liquor present.

e. Decapitation—for obstructed transverse lie with a dead baby. There is a tendency now to recommend Caesarean section instead of decapitation. This is a pity because decapitation is not a difficult operation for an obstetrician with a good pair of hands and a wide experience of intrauterine manoeuvres—forceps delivery for example—even if he has never done decapitation before; for everybody there has to be a first time.

31 Complex Presentation

ARM ALONGSIDE THE HEAD

1. Head above the brim—treat as a transverse lie; it will probably become one.
2. Head in the pelvis—anticipate a normal delivery; if the head can pass the brim with the arm alongside it, it will pass the outlet.

LEG ALONGSIDE THE HEAD

Either (*a*) Pull the leg down and push the head up, *converting it into a breech presentation;* or (*b*) *Caesarean section.*

ARM AND LEG ALONGSIDE THE HEAD

Treat as for Leg alongside the Head

Breech Presentation

TYPES

1. Complete or flexed breech; usually in multigravidae.
2. Frank or extended breech; the usual primigravid breech.
3. Footling
4. Knee presentation } More rare.

AETIOLOGY

At 28 weeks breech presentation is normal, but by 34 weeks the majority of fetuses will present by the vertex, as the centre of gravity has moved nearer to the head end of the baby with development of the fetal skull. Thus, *prematurity* will predispose to breech presentation.

The Extended Legs
This may be the primary factor in the case of the primigravid breech.

Chance
This may be the main factor in the multigravid breech, the fetus presenting by the breech when it had at last grown too large to change its presentation again.

Twin Pregnancy

Hydrocephaly

N.B. Doubts have been cast upon the importance of contracted pelvis as a cause of breech presentation.

POSITIONS

1st position, LSA	3rd position, RSP
2nd position, RSA	4th position, LSP

DIAGNOSIS

Abdominally

Palpation—the absence of the characteristic feel of the head at the brim is the main point. (Auscultation gives no real help.)

Vaginally

The anus is characteristic.

Radiology

This may settle the occasional difficult diagnosis.

MECHANISM

The buttocks, shoulders and head have to be considered separately.

Sacro-anterior Positions

Buttocks (Bitrochanteric Diameter)
1. *Descent.*
2. *Internal Rotation.* One-eighth of a circle.
3. *Lateral Flexion* of the trunk for the birth of the buttocks, anterior first.
4. *Restitution.* One-eighth of a circle in opposite direction to internal rotation.

Shoulders (Bisacromial Diameter)
1. *Descent.*
2. *Internal Rotation.* One-eighth of a circle.
3. *Lateral Flexion* of the neck for delivery of the shoulder.

4. *Restitution.* One-eighth of a circle in opposite direction to internal rotation.

Head (Suboccipito- or Occipitofrontal Diameter)

1. *Descent.*

2. *Internal Rotation.* One-eighth of a circle.

3. Chin, face, brow and vertex sweep over the perineum

Sacro-posterior Positions

Buttocks   As above.

Shoulders

1. *Descent.*

2. *Internal Rotation.* One-eighth of a circle.

Long Internal Rotation of Head	*Short Internal Rotation of Head*
3. Instead of restituting, the *Rotation continues in the same direction* for a further two-eighths of a circle (making the occiput rotate forwards into an anterior position).	*Restitution.* One-eighth of a circle in the opposite direction to internal rotation.

Head

Long Internal Rotation	*Short Internal Rotation*
1. *Descent.* **2.** *Internal Rotation* of three-eighths of a circle, carrying the occiput under the pubic arch. **3.** Chin, face, brow and vertex sweep over the perineum.	*Descent.* *Internal Rotation.* One eighth of a circle, carrying occiput into the hollow of the sacrum. Occiput, vertex, brow, and face sweep over the perineum. *N.B.* This mechanism is most undesirable, but fortunately rare.

RISKS

Maternal

Should not be increased compared with normal vertex delivery:
1. Episiotomy
2. Anaesthesia   More frequent

Fetal

Fetal Loss. Higher than with vertex delivery in most centres, e.g. 7% as compared with 2% would be a not unreasonable assessment and there is no significant difference between multigravidae and primigravidae*.

Essential Difference between breech and vertex delivery from the fetal points of view:
a. In vertex delivery, the head can take 24 hours or more to mould through the pelvis gradually.
b. In breech delivery, it must pass in 7 minutes or the baby will be lost. When the umbilicus has escaped from the vulva, the head is entering the brim with the cord alongside as it passes from umbilicus to placenta and will be *pressed on by the head*. Moreover, after the body has been born the considerable retraction that takes place may cause the *placenta to separate*. The fetus is therefore exposed to the risk of too rapid delivery with cerebral haemorrhage on the one hand, or too slow delivery with asphyxia on the other. The former is the greater risk.

Causes of Fetal Loss
1. *Cerebral Haemorrhage* due to the rapid moulding necessary to deliver the baby within the 7 minutes. This is the commonest accident. Therefore use as much of the 7 minutes as possible.
2. *Failure to Deliver the Baby within 7 Minutes.* This is rare except with:
a. Contracted pelvis—if the pelvis is contracted, the baby must be delivered abdominally.

*Redman T. F. (1950) *Br. Med. J.* **1**, 814.

b. An unexpected delivery and *no attendant present.*
c. Cervical dystocia when the relatively small body of a premature fetus slips through the undilated cervix and the head cannot follow.
d. Extended arms.

3. *Prolapse of the Cord.* Six times more common in breech than vertex presentation due to:
a. A badly fitting presenting part.
b. Umbilicus being nearer the most dependent point.

Contra-indication to Vaginal Delivery in Breech Presentation
1. Contracted pelvis.
2. Primigravidae over 35 years of age.
3. A large baby, e.g. > 8 lb (3630 g) but this is difficult to judge.
N.B.   There is a growing tendency to perform Caesarean section almost routinely for breech presentation to avoid the admittedly slightly higher fetal loss with vaginal delivery. However, this loss can be kept to a minimum if all breech deliveries are done or supervised by experienced obstetricians. Moreover, it must be remembered that Caesarean section carries a maternal death rate due to the operation itself of 0·8 per 1000 operations (*Report on Confidential Enquiries into Maternal Deaths in England and Wales, 1976–1978*).

MANAGEMENT

Pregnancy

External Version without anaesthesia. Anaesthesia is seldom used now but it may have a small place where there is a contracted pelvis and the alternative would be a Caesarean section electively, but be cautious (*see below*).

1. *Contra-indication to External Version for Breech Presentation*

a. Antepartum haemorrhage

b. A case where elective Caesarean section is contemplated regardless of the presentation

c. Twins

d. Abnormal or dead fetus

⎫ Absolute contra-indica-tions ⎬

e. Pre-eclampsia, essential hypertension, or chronic nephritis—relative factors.

2. *Optimum Time is 34 Weeks*

a. Less than this and the presentation may recur (but sometimes it is wise to do it at 32 weeks—if it is easy nothing is lost).

b. Later than this may be leaving it too late for success but—it is never too late to try, and a few cases may still undergo spontaneous version, even where version has failed under anaesthesia.

3. *Dangers of Version.* These mostly apply to version under anaesthesia.

a. Separation of placenta with death of the baby, i.e. accidental haemorrhage.

b. Premature labour.

c. Abnormal lie or attitude of the fetus which cannot be corrected, e.g. 'a flying fetus'.

d. Rupture of the uterus.

e. Transplacental bleeding (fetomaternal). Anti-D antiserum is often advised in Rh-negative women after attempted version.

4. *Fetal Loss due to External Version*

a. Without anaesthesia: negligible.

b. With anaesthesia: 2% is a low figure.

N.B. The anaesthesia must be used only to obtain relaxation and not to allow great force to be used. Warn the patient *beforehand* that it may not succeed and that breech delivery is not a cause for alarm; then the operator is less likely to persist against his better judgement.

5. The evidence that a policy of performing cephalic version reduces the incidence of breech delivery is equivocal; some say that where it succeeds spontaneous version would have occurred anyway. Nevertheless, it is still widely performed, and without anaesthesia, at least, it is harmless.

Assess the Pelvis, radiographically in the primigravida and where necessary in the multigravida, otherwise by vaginal examination. *This must be always done regardless of the size of previous babies.*

Assisted Breech Delivery

The management of labour until this point has no special features.

Preparations
1. An obstetrician and an anaesthetist must be in the labour ward at the beginning of delivery.
2. A *forceps trolley* is required to include:
a. A pudendal block set.
b. Lignocaine (Xylocaine) 1%.
c. Simpson–Barnes or Wrigley's forceps.
d. Episiotomy scissors.
3. *Anaesthetic Apparatus* ready prepared for a 'crash' induction if required.

Lithotomy Position and towel off as for forceps delivery.

Catheterize

Episiotomy under local anaesthesia, as the anus appears over the perineum, in all primigravidae, and, where necessary, in multigravidae.
N.B. Do not do it too early or blood may be lost before the breech distends the vulva.

Do not exert Traction on the Breech at any time or arms and head may be swept up and become extended. As far as possible the baby should be pushed out by the mother.
The *only* occasions when the baby should be *touched during delivery* are to:
1. *Assist the Feet over the Perineum* in an extended breech, by flexing the knees out to the flank.

2. *Pull Down a Loop of Cord* when the umbilicus appears, to prevent traction on it.

3. *Bring Down the Arms,* if they do not come down spontaneously, by sweeping the elbows across the baby's face.

4. *Deliver the Head.* The following methods are available:

a. Mauriceau–Smellie–Veit. Jaw and shoulder traction.

b. Wigand–Martin. Jaw and shoulder traction with one hand and suprapubic pressure with the other.

c. Forceps. Best method, especially for the primigravida.

d. Burns–Marshall or Liverpool. Allow the baby to hang by the head to bring it into the pelvis and deliver it by sweeping the body over the pubis, holding the feet in the left hand, exerting some traction, and controlling the perineum with the right hand.

N.B. Although a special point of letting the baby hang is made in the Liverpool method, it is advocated for general use whatever method is used for delivering the head. A rapid induction of anaesthesia may be required for delivery of the head, although local analgesia is usually enough.

Management of Complications

Failure of Breech to Descend

1. *Groin Traction* with the forefinger on the extended breech, but only during a contraction and while the mother pushes.

2. *Breech Extraction,* under epidural or general anaesthesia, bringing down the legs in the case of the extended breech.

3. *Blunt Hook,* only on a dead baby and if the legs are extended.

Extended Arms

1. Løvset's manoeuvre.

2. Bring down the arms under full anaesthesia.

Arrest of the Head at the Brim (Disproportion or Extended Head)   Bring it

through the brim under full anaesthesia by the Mauriceau–Smellie–Veit manoeuvre, or Wigand–Martin manoeuvre. The head is brought through the brim in the transverse position and then rotated one-quarter of a circle in the pelvic cavity before extraction.

If anaesthesia is not available, the Wigand–Martin manoeuvre is the only possible procedure.

N.B.   An unsuspected hydrocephalus may lead to the head not passing the brim.

Diagnosis: (1) Wide sutures in the temporal and occipital region; (2) There may be a lumbar spina bifida.

Treatment: Perforation of the head through the occiput, running up a pair of sharp-pointed scissors subcutaneously.

After-coming Head Occipitoposterior
1. Attempt to rotate the chin posteriorly, or
2. Deliver chin to the front by:
a. Van Hoorn's manoeuvre (shoulder traction from behind and suprapubic pressure) or
b. Forceps.

Multiple Pregnancy

INCIDENCE

Twins	1 in 80 births
Triplets	1 in 80 × 80 = 6400 births
Quadruplets	1 in 80 × 80 × 80 = 512000 births

TYPES

	Binovular	*Uniovular*
Origin	Two ova from 1 or 2 follicles	1 ovum
Incidence	75%	25%
Sexes	May be opposite sex	Same sex
Chorion	Two separate ones	One only
Circulation	Separate	May communicate

HEREDITY

Binovular twinning has a familial tendency and this can be on the father's as well as the mother's side.

Uniovular twinning is a chance occurrence except after induced ovulation.

FREQUENCY OF COMBINATION OF PRESENTING PART

First Baby	Second Baby	Per Cent
Vertex	Vertex	40
Vertex	Breech	20
Breech	Vertex	15
Breech	Breech	10
Vertex	Transverse	8
Breech	Transverse	4
Transverse	Vertex	1
Transverse	Breech	1
Transverse	Transverse	1

DIAGNOSIS

Method of Presenting Clinically

1. Routine ultrasound examination between 14 and 20 weeks (especially likely in cases where pregnancy resulted after induced ovulation).
2. Polyhydramnios: Tense uterus with fluid thrill.
3. Uterus large for the period of gestation.
a. The bulk of two fetuses, or
b. Hydramnios (*see above*)
4. Palpation of two fetuses.
a. Three or more fetal poles.
b. Multiple limbs and no easily palpable back.
c. Fetal head small for size of uterine contents.

Confirmatory Methods

1. X-ray or ultrasound.
2. Detection of two separate fetal hearts.
a. Two observers listening simultaneously, and
b. Count for one minute, and
c. A difference of at least 10 between the rates.

EFFECTS

Upon Pregnancy

1. Polyhydramnios.
a. Maternal discomfort, abdominal pain, oedema of legs and dyspnoea in pregnancy.
b. Prolapsed cord when membranes rupture.
2. Pre-eclampsia and eclampsia are more common.
3. Placenta praevia (due to size of the placenta).
4. Premature labour.
5. Anaemia—both megaloblastic and iron-deficiency.

Upon Labour

1. Malpresentations.
a. Transverse lie, especially of 2nd twin.
b. Locked twins:
i. Breech—vertex.
ii. Vertex—vertex.
2. Prolapsed cord.
a. Polyhydramnios.
b. Transverse lie.
3. Premature separation of placenta of 2nd child due to uterine shrinkage after birth of 1st baby.
4. Postpartum haemorrhage (due to large placental site).
N.B. Inertia in the 1st and 2nd stages is not more common in multiple pregnancy (Jeffcoate), although it is often stated to the contrary.

PROGNOSIS

Causes of Maternal Death

1. Postpartum haemorrhage.
2. Operative interference for malpresentation; sepsis, inhalation pneumonia, shock, etc.
3. Pre-eclampsia and eclampsia, q.v.

Causes of Fetal Death

1. Prematurity.
2. Separation of 2nd placenta after delivery of 1st child.
3. Malpresentation, particularly of the 2nd child.
4. Prolapsed cord.
5. Pre-eclampsia and eclampsia.

N.B. It is the second child that is at risk mainly.

MANAGEMENT

Pregnancy

1. Ensure considerable rest between 28 and 36 weeks, resting in bed, perhaps in hospital, from the 28th to the 30th week, to prevent premature labour. The evidence from controlled studies, however, does not demonstrate any improvement in fetal salvage by this method of management.
2. Adequate diet, with supplements of iron and folic acid.
3. Insomnia may be troublesome later in pregnancy.
4. Always book for hospital confinement.

Labour

As for any labour until after delivery of first child, then proceed as follows:
1. Palpate abdomen to find lie of 2nd fetus; if it is transverse make it longitudinal, preferably vertex, by external version.
2. Listen to fetal heart rate.
3. Tie cord of delivery infant on maternal as well as on fetal side (danger of communicating circulation).
4. If no further contractions within 10 min of delivering baby:
a. Perform a vaginal examination.
b. Rupture forewaters of 2nd fetus and keep examining fingers in cervix until the presenting part descends into pelvis, to diagnose prolapsed cord.

5. If second baby is not likely to join first within half an hour, the doctor should deliver it.

6. Ergometrine with the anterior shoulder of the second baby, intravenously.

Complications with Second Baby

Indications for Delivery of Second Baby
1. Prolapsed cord.
2. Transverse lie.
3. Failure to get two babies in the cot within half an hour of each other.
4. Fetal distress.

Methods of Delivery
1. Head in pelvis—forceps.
2. Head above brim or transverse lie—internal version and breech extraction.
3. Breech presenting—breech extraction.

DEFINITIONS

Presentation of the Cord

A loop of cord lies below the presenting part but the membranes are intact.

Prolapse of the Cord

A loop of cord lies below the presenting part and the membranes have ruptured.

Occult Prolapse of the Cord

A loop of cord lies alongside the presenting part, after rupture of the membranes, and is subject to pressure. It may not be palpable on vaginal examination.

CAUSES

Badly-fitting Presenting Part

Faults in the Fetus
1. Breech.
2. Transverse lie (including the second of twins).
3. Posterior position.

Faults in the Pelvis
1. Flat pelvis.
2. Tumours in or of the pelvis.

Very High Presenting Part

1. Multiparity.
2. Polyhydramnios.

DIAGNOSIS

1. By vaginal examination, performed:
a. As a routine when the membranes rupture; or
b. For some other purpose in the course of labour, prolapsed cord being an accidental discovery; or
c. On account of marked alteration of the fetal heart rate with each uterine contraction.
2. Cord appears at vulva.

N.B. A vaginal examination should be made within a matter of minutes when the membranes rupture in the presence of a high presenting part.

TREATMENT

By the Midwife, if the Baby be Alive

1. If near delivery, achieve this as quickly as possible, helped by an episiotomy.
2. If not near delivery:
a. Send for medical aid, and
b. Prevent pressure on the cord by:
Either: (i) Keeping the fingers in the vagina either between the presenting part and the pelvic brim, protecting the cord, or pressing the presenting part up with each contraction.
Or: (ii) Placing the patient in the genupectoral position (not of much use).

By the Doctor, if the Baby be Alive

1. Deliver the baby as soon as possible—the safest plan:
a. By forceps, or by breech extraction, or
b. By Caesarean section, or
2. Replace the cord with gauze—individual

swabs or a roll of 15-cm gauze. This is liable to be more dangerous to the fetus but may be justified in a 'grand multipara' in whom speedy delivery is expected.

If the Baby be Dead

No special action is required on account of the prolapsed cord: just await spontaneous delivery, if this is anticipated.

35 Inverted Uterus

CAUSES

1. Pressing on the fundus of a flaccid uterus.
2. Pulling on the cord when the placenta is inserted on the fundus and the uterus is flaccid.
3. A fundally inserted placenta with partial morbid adherence.

DIAGNOSIS

Think of the possibility when a patient is *severely shocked,* out of all proportion to the blood loss, after delivery of the baby. A *vaginal examination* will detect the uterine fundus in the vagina.
N.B. It is seldom that the condition can be detected by abdominal examination, although 'dimpling' of the uterine fundus has been described.

PROPHYLAXIS

Proper management of the third stage of labour.

TREATMENT

Acute Puerperal Inversion

Start a *blood drip* and then without waiting further:
1. *Manual Replacement,* or
2. *Hydrostatic Replacement.*
a. Requirements:
  i. Douche-can and rubber tubing.
  ii. Four litres of sterile water or lotion (most of it goes on the floor!).
  iii. Many vulval pads.
b. Technique: The surgeon inserts his hand, holding the end of the rubber tubing into the vagina and attempts to make a seal between his wrist and the vulva using the vulval pads and his other hand. An assistant stands on a chair and pours the sterile fluid into the douche-can, then holds the can up high. The hydrostatic pressure distends the vagina and gradually pushes the uterus back into place.
N.B. The patient will probably not recover from shock until the uterus is replaced.

Chronic Inversion

I.e. a case which has not been diagnosed or treated at delivery—*Aveling's repositor.*

36   Ruptured Uterus

CAUSES

**Spon-
taneous
Rupture**

Obstructed Labour
E.g. shoulder presentation, disproportion, etc.
The lower segment becomes very thin due to
exaggerated retraction of the upper segment
and the formation of Bandl's ring.

Scars from Previous Uterine Operation
1. Caesarean section.
N.B. A placenta implanted under the old
scar weakens it.
2. Myomectomy.
3. Perforation of the uterus with a curette or
dilator.
4. Hysterotomy.

**Misuse of Oxytocics such as Oxytocin or
Ergometrine**

Cases with no Obvious Cause occur
But it is presumed that there had been a
weakened uterus present as the result of
previous unrecognized damage. It is usual to
find, therefore, that the patient:
1. Is multiparous, or
2. Has a history of previous instrumental
vaginal delivery.

N.B.   Spontaneous rupture seldom occurs in a primigravid patient because:
a. The uterus is less weakened and is unscarred, except when there has been a previous operation.
b. If obstruction occurs, the uterus tends to act inefficiently which protects it from rupture.

Traumatic Rupture

Internal Version
When the lower segment has thinned too much and there is inadequate liquor present (the commonest cause).

Forceps Delivery
When the cervix has not reached full dilatation.

PATHOLOGY

Types of Tear

A tear may be *complete* (into the peritoneal cavity) or *incomplete* (into the broad ligament).

Site of Tear

1. *Vertically up the Lateral Wall,* usually starting as a tear of the cervix; *'spontaneous ruptures with no obvious cause'* and *'traumatic ruptures'* are usually of this type. The uterine vessels may be torn, and haemorrhage and shock severe.
2. *Vertically up the Anterior Wall.* Rupture of a *classic Caesarean section scar.*
3. *Horizontal Tear of the Lower Segment.* Rupture:
a. After obstructed labour.
b. After misuse of oxytocin.
c. Of a lower segment Caesarean section scar.
   Some scars, e.g. lower segment Caesarean section one, may *herniate* gradually before ultimate rupture.

CLINICAL PICTURE

Acute Rupture

1. Severe shock.
2. Abdominal pain and tenderness—sudden in onset: it feels as though 'something has given way'.
3. Vaginal bleeding.
4. If the baby has not been born:
   a. Uterine contractions ⎫ will have
   b. Fetal heart sounds ⎬ disappeared.
   ⎭

Subacute Rupture

1. No shock.
2. Abdominal pain and tenderness is less.
3. The bleeding is slight.
4. The fetal heart may still be heard.

'Silent' Rupture

1. A *suprapubic bulge* may herald herniation through a lower segment Caesarean section scar. The bulge persists despite catheterization.
2. A spontaneous rupture may occasionally occur with no immediate symptoms: presumably an old scar has given way gradually and bloodlessly. *Simultaneous cessation of both uterine contractions and the fetal heart sound* indicates such an accident.

PROPHYLAXIS

1. Early recognition of obstructed labour.
N.B. Be very watchful when full dilatation has been passed in multiparae; never leave her for more than 1 hour in the second stage. However, disproportion does not increase the strain across the lower segment over what is to be expected in any labour until the head is clamped into the brim by the uterine action.
2. Admit certain cases to hospital before labour begins:
a. Previous classic Caesarean section or myomectomy (1 week before term).

b. Unstable lie once 38 weeks has been reached.

3. Confine the 'grand multipara' in hospital.

4. Take great care in the control of oxytocin infusions (*see* pp. 229 and 296).

TREATMENT

At Home   Anti-shock treatment and send for the 'Flying Squad'.

In Hospital   **1.** Resuscitation by blood transfusion, on the theatre table preferably; then,

2. Laparotomy and:

a. Remove the uterus (as well as the baby, etc., if still present), or

b. Repair the rent.

37 Obstetrical Operations

VERSION

External Version

1. *Definition: External Cephalic Version* is to correct a transverse lie or breech presentation to a vertex presentation by manipulation through the abdominal wall.

2. *Contra-indications*
3. *Optimum Time*
4. *Dangers*
5. *Fetal Mortality*
⎫ *See under* 'Breech Presentation',
⎬ Chapter 32.
⎭

Bipolar Version

1. *Definition.* The right hand is inserted into the vagina and two fingers into the uterus. The left hand placed on the abdomen brings the breech, and hence a foot, within reach of the two fingers within the uterus; seize the foot and draw it out through the vulva.

2. *Sequel.* Breech delivery.

3. *Use*

a. To convert a transverse lie into a breech presentation.

b. To control bleeding from a minor degree of placenta praevia by plugging the lower segment with the half-breech. (Now only used if the baby is dead, abnormal, or too small for a reasonable chance of survival.)

Internal Version

1. *Definition.* The whole hand is inserted into the uterus and a foot grasped and brought down.
2. *Sequelae*
a. Breech delivery, or
b. Breech extraction.
3. *Use*
a. To correct a transverse lie.
b. To deliver a case with a floating head, e.g. second of twins; brow presentation.
N.B.   This manoeuvre can only be performed safely for mother and baby if there is still adequate liquor present and the uterus has not begun to mould around the baby. If it is attempted without these conditions being fulfilled, the uterus will rupture and the baby will probably be killed or badly injured.

FORCEPS DELIVERY

History of the Obstetric Forceps

1720	*Palfryn* of Ghent. First published description. A pair of spoon-shaped blades with wood handles and tied with string.
1600 (approx.)	The *Chamberlen family,* starting with Peter Chamberlen, were using forceps in a fashionable London practice but it was kept a family secret and only became generally known about 100 years later. In 1818, 3 pairs of forceps were found in a chest in a house once owned by the Chamberlens; 2 pairs had a pin at the fulcrum and one used tape. The last of the line, Hugh Chamberlen (junior), died in 1728 and he is commemorated by a plaque in Westminster Abbey.
1746	*William Smellie* described the *English lock.* He also lengthened the shank to 2½ in.

1747	*Levret* described the pelvic curve to the Paris Academy.
1877	*Tarnier* of Paris—described axis traction forceps.
1914	*Kielland*—described his instrument

Indications

There are many, but all resolve eventually into cases of incipient or actual fetal or maternal distress.

Conditions which must be fulfilled before attempting Forceps Delivery

1. Fully dilated cervix.
2. Forceps must only be applied to the fetal head and a suitable position of the head must be present at delivery, e.g.:
   a. Occipito-anterior position of the vertex.
   b. Mento-anterior position of the face.
   c. Aftercoming head of the breech with the occiput under the pubic arch.
   d. Occipitoposterior positions of the vertex (undesirable as a rule).
   N.B.   Forceps are *never* applied to:
   a. Brow presentation
   b. Mentoposterior position of the face
   c. A lateral position of the head (vertex or face), except Kielland's forceps
   d. The breech
   } Unless first corrected to a suitable presentation and position (*see below*).
3. The head must be engaged.
4. There must be no gross outlet disproportion.
5. The membranes must be ruptured.

Dangers

To the Mother
1. Tears of cervix or vagina.
2. Infection.
3. Mendelson's syndrome and inhalation pneumonia if a general anaesthetic is used (*see* pp. 186, 225 and 298).

4. Postpartum haemorrhage; effect of general anaesthetic on the uterus.
N.B. Pudendal block and epidural anaesthesia have to a great extent replaced general anaesthesia for suitable cases of forceps delivery, with increased safety to mother and baby.

To the Baby
1. Intracranial haemorrhage.
2. Asphyxia neonatorum due to general anaesthesia.

Method of Dealing with Lateral or Oblique Positions of the Fetal Head

1. Manual rotation.
2. Forceps rotation by Kielland's forceps.

Types of Forceps in General Use

1. Simpson's. Serrated handle, but no knees.
2. Barnes's. Knees, but a smooth handle.
3. Simpson–Barnes's. Serrated handle and knees. Also known as Anderson's.
4. Neville–Barnes's. Barnes's forceps with an axis-traction attachment to the handle.
N.B. Simpson–Barnes's forceps with the Neville axis traction attachment are more popular and generally useful.
5. Milne–Murray's. True axis traction.
6. Kielland's. No pelvic curve and has a sliding lock.
7. Wrigley's. Delicate blades with a small handle.

VACUUM EXTRACTION OR VENTOUSE DELIVERY

Indications   As for forceps delivery

Conditions under which Delivery may be considered

Although vacuum extraction may be considered as an alternative to forceps extraction, and in some centres it is so employed, there may be a greater place for its use where forceps application would normally be prohibited, e.g.:
1. Before full dilatation, or
2. When the head is not fully engaged.
In such cases the cervix may become fully dilated or the head brought low enough by the venthouse to effect delivery by vacuum extraction or to complete the delivery safely by forceps. Such a manoeuvre must be done in the labour-room theatre with facilities for Caesarean section immediately available.

Advantages

1. Anaesthesia is not necessarily required.
2. Used with discretion it should be safe a technique for mother and baby.
3. It may be useful in cases such as those just described, where forceps would be contra-indicated.

Dis-advantages

1. It is not so effective as the forceps where rotation is required.
2. It is more time-consuming than forceps delivery (it takes 6–8 min to reach an effective vacuum before beginning traction).
3. If a hard pull is required, the cup will pull off (this may also be a protection).
4. The vacuum raises an exaggerated 'caput' on the scalp, called a 'chignon'. This subsides considerably in a few hours but may take several days to go completely. It is ugly but has no serious implications.

Technique

Three sizes of cup are supplied: the largest which can be applied is used.
  The vacuum is created by a hand 'pump'. The degree of vacuum is recorded on a dial and is raised to 0·6 or 0·8 kg/sq cm in stages

of 0·2 kg/sq cm every 2 min, i.e. it takes 6–8 min to reach full vacuum.

Traction is exerted during contractions. The time to effect delivery is variable, but if not achieved within 30 min it should be abandoned: it should be exceptional to try even so long.

EPISIOTOMY

Indications

1. To prevent severe laceration with:
a. An inelastic perineum.
b. Face-to-pubes delivery.
c. Face delivery.
d. A narrow pubic arch.
e. Previous third-degree tear repair.
f. Previous colpoperineorrhaphy.
2. To facilitate delivery where the delay on the perineum is too long for the mother's tolerance or the baby's safety.
3. Breech delivery; for the aftercoming head in most primigravidae and many multigravidae.
4. Premature labour to avoid cerebral damage.
5. To achieve quick delivery in cases of:
a. Fetal distress.
b. Cardiac disease.
c. Prolapsed cord.

Technique

1. Local anaesthesia should *always* be used unless epidural analgesia is present.
2. Two types are acceptable:
a. Mediolateral: starting at the fourchette and running out obliquely.
b. J-shaped: starting in the midline, then curving outwards.

Breakdown of Episiotomy or a Tear in the Puerperium

Do not Resuture. Let it heal spontaneously wearing a pad as long as is necessary. The end result when seen at the postnatal clinic will show little evidence of the breakdown.

Reasons for not Resuturing
1. Resuture has a 50% incidence of further breakdown.

2. There is less discomfort if not resutured than if it is.

3. The end result is better if left to heal with less chance of (i) dyspareunia; (ii) a tear in a future labour (cf. p. 194).

CAESAREAN SECTION

Types

Lower Segment Caesarean Section

1. This is the form which is now almost universally performed, where it is possible to do so.

2. It is a transverse incision in the lower segment after pushing down the bladder.

Upper Segment Caesarean Section (Classic CS)

1. This is very seldom performed, the main indications being:

a. A fibroid occupying the lower segment.

b. A shoulder presentation impacted into the pelvis.

2. It is a vertical midline incision in the upper segment anterior wall.

3. *Dangers*

a. Rupture is more likely in a subsequent pregnancy than it is after the lower segment operation, and if rupture occurs it is usually more disastrous (*see under* 'Ruptured Uterus', Chapter 36). The reasons for this greater tendency to rupture are: (1) The upper segment stretches more than the lower during subsequent pregnancy, (2) The scar is weaker because: (i) it is a fibrous union between two great thicknesses of muscle; (ii) the upper segment is not at rest in the puerperium. (3) The placenta may be inserted under it, eroding into and weakening it.

b. Adhesions are more likely to form, giving rise to strangulations, etc.

METHODS OF TERMINATING PREGNANCY

Twelve Weeks or Under

Evacuate with:
1. The Kerslake suction evacuator (best method).
2. Dilators and ovum forceps.

Over Twelve Weeks and under Twenty-eight Weeks

No method is without some danger.
1. Abdominal hysterotomy (considerable danger of rupture in subsequent pregnancies).
2. Prostaglandin
a. Intra-amniotic Prostaglandin $F_{2\alpha}$ 8 ml (5 mg/ml) injected slowly into the amniotic sac.
b. Extra-amniotic Prostaglandin E_2. (i) A 12–14 French gauge Foley catheter is inserted extra-amniotically. (ii) A diluted solution containing 100 mg/ml is prepared. (*a*) Initial instillation—1 ml; (*b*) Further instillation—1–2 ml at 2-hourly intervals, according to the response.
An i.v. infusion of oxytocin can be used to supplement prostaglandins if necessary.
3. Aretus or Utus paste (dangerous).
4. Introduction of hydrostatic bag—Taylor's or Queen Charlotte's (danger of sepsis, only of historic interest.).

Twenty-eight Weeks or Over

1. A *Prostaglandin pessary* or *prostaglandin gel* is inserted the night before induction is planned. Near term labour may start with this alone.
2. Artificial rupture of membranes.
a. Hindwater puncture (Drew-Smythe catheter) or
b. Forewater rupture.
This is usually done early in the day.
3. *Oxytocin* (Syntocinon is the synthetic preparation used). Little use on its own but is

used to increase the efficiency of surgical induction (*see* p. 229 for details).

When used for induction the dosage can be raised to higher levels. This is safe when stimulating inefficient uterine action, but once the uterus begins to respond the dosage may have to be cut back quickly as one may well then be stimulating a normal uterine action with dire consequences, such as uterine rupture.

4. *Caesarean Section* is likely to be used the earlier in pregnancy delivery is planned, especially under 34 weeks. Increasingly, more premature deliveries are being undertaken, for with modern techniques the paediatricians have such good results with very premature babies.

DESTRUCTIVE OPERATIONS

N.B. These are only applied to *dead* or *abnormal babies.*

Operations for Reducing the Size of the Fetal Head

Simple Perforation of the Hydrocephalic Head to release cerebrospinal fluid and allow the head to be born.

1. *Forecoming Head.* Drive a *pair of long, sharp-pointed scissors* through a fontanelle or wide suture, open the blades and allow the cerebrospinal fluid to flow. Do not remove the blades till it has all escaped. The head will descend into the pelvis at once.

2. *Aftercoming Head.* Pick up the skin at the nape of the neck with a pair of *toothed dissecting forceps,* make a cut with a pair of *long, sharp-pointed scissors* and then drive them up subcutaneously to the occipital region, perforating, and allowing the cerebrospinal fluid to run off. The head will now deliver easily.

Perforation and Crushing of the skull in a

dead baby when delivery is held up by disproportion, abnormal presentation (e.g. brow), or a cervix not fully dilated.

1. Perforate the skull with *Simpson's perforator* (craniotomy).

2. Crush the skull with a *three-bladed, combined cranioclast and cephalotribe,* and extract.

Decapitation for Obstructed Transverse Lie and a Dead Baby	**1.** Decapitate with *Jardine's decapitation knife.* **2.** Deliver the body. **3.** Deliver the head using a finger in the mouth or a *crotchet* inserted inside the skull.
Cleidotomy	The division of both clavicles when the shoulders become arrested with a very large baby. Use *cleidotomy scissors*—long handles and short blades.
Evisceration and Bifurcation	These are the means of dealing with dystocia caused by tumours or monsters.
Summary of Instruments required for Destructive Operations	(In addition to a normal forceps trolley) Simpson's perforator. Three-bladed combined cranioclast and cephalotribe. Jardine's decapitation knife. Crotchet and blunt hook. Cleidotomy scissors. A pair of lateral vaginal wall retractors. Auvard's speculum. Vulsellum forceps—4. Ferguson's scissors. Douche can and nozzle.

PREPARATION FOR GENERAL ANAESTHESIA

For patients in late pregnancy or labour before leaving the ward:

1. Pass a nasogastric tube.

2. Give Mist. Mag. Trisil. 15 ml.

These precautions are to reduce the risk of death from Mendelson's Syndrome (*see* pp. 186, 225 and 290).

Appendix **Obstetric Mortality Statistics**

DEFINITIONS

All these rates are expressed as a ratio of 1000 total (live and still) births, except the neonatal mortality rate, which is related only to live births.
From 1983 the **Maternal Mortality Rate** is expressed as a ratio of 100 000 total (live and still) births and the **Stillbirth Rate** as a ratio of 100 total (live and still) births.

Maternal Mortality Rate

(Excluding abortion since 1941 in the Registrar-General's return). The number of maternal deaths associated with pregnancy and child-bearing per 1000 total (live and still) births (100 000 from 1983).

Stillbirth Rate

The number of stillbirths per 1000 total (live and still) births (100 from 1983).

Neonatal Mortality Rate

The number of deaths in the first 4 weeks of life per 1000 registered live births.

299

Perinatal Mortality Rate

The number of stillbirths together with the early neonatal deaths (deaths in the first week of life) per 1000 total (live and still) births.

This latter rate is the best index of the loss of life due to antenatal and obstetric factors, deaths at a late time being more likely to result from postnatal events.

VITAL STATISTICS FOR ENGLAND AND WALES

	1964	1972	1982	1983	
Maternal Mortality Rate					
Maternal causes, excluding abortion	0·20	0·12	0·083	7·1	(per 100000 total births)
Total maternal mortality	0·25	0·15	0·09	8·4	(per 100000 total births)
Stillbirth Rate	16·4	12	6·3	0·57	(per 100 total births)
Neonatal Mortality Rate	13·8	12	6·3	5·9	
Perinatal Mortality Rate	28·2	22	11·3	10·4	

since 1983

Index